BAD FAITH

Also by Paul A. Offit, M.D.

Deadly Choices

Vaccinated

The Cutter Incident

Autism's False Prophets

Do You Believe in Magic?

BAD FAITH

When Religious Belief Undermines Modern Medicine

PAUL A. OFFIT, M.D.

BASIC BOOKS

A Member of the Perseus Books Group

New York

Published by Basic Books, A Member of the Perseus Books Group

Books published by Basic Books are available at special discounts for bulk purchases in the United States by corporations, institutions, and other organizations. For more information, please contact the Special Markets Department at the Perseus Books Group, 2300 Chestnut Street, Suite 200, Philadelphia, PA 19103, or call (800) 810-4145, ext. 5000, or e-mail special.markets@perseusbooks.com.

Design by Cynthia Young in Adobe Garamond Pro

Library of Congress Cataloging-in-Publication Data
Offit, Paul A., author.
    Bad faith : when religious belief undermines modern medicine / Paul A. Offit.
        p. ; cm.
    Includes bibliographical references and index.
    ISBN 978-0-465-08296-4 (hardcover)—ISBN 978-0-465-04061-2 (e-book)
    I. Title.
    [DNLM: 1. Religion and Medicine.   2. Child Welfare.   3. Faith Healing.
    4. Treatment Refusal.   BL 65.M4]
    BL65.M4
    201.661—dc23

                                                            2014041626

10 9 8 7 6 5 4 3 2 1

To all those who perform good deeds
in the name of their faith

Verily, I say unto you,
Inasmuch as you have done it unto
one of the least of my brethren
you have done it unto me.

—Matthew 25:40

CONTENTS

INTRODUCTION:
AT THE CROSSROADS

"I went down to the crossroads, fell down on my knees.
Asked the Lord above for mercy, 'Save me, if you please.'"

—ROBERT JOHNSON

On April 13, 2013, Brandon Schaible, the seven-month-old son of Herbert and Catherine Schaible, died. For several days, Brandon had suffered from pneumonia. The Schaibles prayed, but to no avail. At 8:00 P.M., they called caretakers at the John F. Fluery & Sons Funeral Home, who called the county medical examiner, who called the police. Paramedics rushed to the house and pronounced the child dead.

It wasn't the first time the Schaibles had lost a child to a treatable illness. A few years earlier, in 2009, the Schaibles had also chosen prayer instead of antibiotics for their two-year-old son, Kent, when he contracted bacterial pneumonia.

Herbert and Catherine Schaible are members of the First-Century Gospel Church, a faith healing group in northeast Philadelphia that relies on the advice given in James 5:14–15: *Is anyone among you sick? Let him call the elders of the church to pray over him and anoint him with oil in the name of the Lord. And the prayer offered in faith will make the sick person well.* After Kent died, Herbert said, "We tried to fight the Devil, but the Devil won."

Every year, tens of thousands of Americans refuse medical care for their children in the name of God.

IN 2009, A SEVENTEEN-YEAR-OLD girl was admitted to a hospital in northeastern Pennsylvania with severe anemia. The doctor told her parents that she needed a blood transfusion to survive. Because the girl and her parents were Jehovah's Witnesses, they refused, quoting Leviticus 7:26: *And wherever you live, you must not eat the blood of any bird or animal.* The doctor got a court order to allow the transfusion that saved her life.

Four years later, the patient, now married and twenty-one years old, returned to the hospital. She wanted to tell a group of medical students not to make the same mistake on other Jehovah's Witnesses that her doctor had made on her. Intelligent, well-spoken, and attractive, with long brown hair and a disarmingly calm demeanor, she stood in front of a group of stunned students and explained how eternal paradise could no longer be hers. "I would rather have died pure," she said, "than to live impure." So moving was her speech that several medical students said that, if confronted with a similar situation, they wouldn't give a blood transfusion.

ON AUGUST 22, 2003, Ray Hemphill, an evangelist at the Faith Temple Church of Apostolic Faith in Milwaukee, performed an exorcism on Terrance Cottrell Jr., an eight-year-old boy with autism. Hemphill quoted Mark 1:25–26: *'Be quiet!' said Jesus sternly. 'Come out of him!' The impure spirit shook the man violently and came out of him with a shriek.*

Hemphill placed Terrance on the floor, put his knee on the boy's chest, and screamed, "In the name of Jesus, Devil get out!" Two hours later, Terrance Cottrell Jr. was dead. The coroner reported that Terrance had died from "mechanical asphyxiation due to external chest compression."

In 2005, in response to growing demand, a pontifical academy in Rome sponsored an exorcism training course in Baltimore; more than a hundred priests and bishops showed up.

IN NOVEMBER 2004, New York City's Department of Health received a report about two newborn boys from Brooklyn who had suffered herpes virus infections. Both had been circumcised by the same ultra-Orthodox Jewish *mohel* (person who performs a ritual circumcision), who pointed to a sixteenth-century religious text stating that after performing a circumcision, *We spit blood into the earth*.

Eight years later, on June 8, 2012, Centers for Disease Control and Prevention (CDC) researchers traveled to New York City to investigate another herpes outbreak. This time it wasn't two babies who'd been infected with herpes; it was eleven. Two of the eleven had died, and two others had suffered permanent brain damage. All had been circumcised by *mohels* who had used their mouths to suck off the blood. New York City health officials estimate that the procedure, called *metzitzah b'peh* (sucking with the mouth), is performed on about thirty-six hundred babies in their city every year—and on tens of thousands throughout the world.

ON AUGUST 14, 2013, sixteen people in Tarrant County, Texas—including a four-month-old infant—came down with measles. A few days later, another five children from nearby Denton County also developed measles. All of the cases were traced to the Eagle Mountain International Church, a ministry associated with a popular televangelist named Kenneth Copeland. Measles had spread through the congregation, the staff, and a daycare center on church property. Virtually everyone who became infected was unvaccinated.

During the outbreak, churchgoers were unafraid "'cause I know Jesus is a healer," said one. "So I know that He's covered us with His blood." More than a thousand people in the surrounding community were exposed in what became the largest measles outbreak in the United States in more than twenty years. Frightened, church officials immediately encouraged parishioners to get their measles vaccine.

On any given day in America, tens of thousands of children whose parents have chosen not to vaccinate them for religious reasons can be found in daycare centers, schools, playgrounds, and churches across the country.

ON NOVEMBER 3, 2009, a twenty-seven-year-old mother of four entered St. Joseph's Medical Center, a Roman Catholic hospital in Phoenix, Arizona. The woman was eleven weeks pregnant and gravely ill, suffering from a disorder called pulmonary hypertension. Because the arterial pressure in her lungs was extremely high, the right side of her heart, which pumps blood to the lungs, had begun to fail. Badly. The problem had been caused by her pregnancy. For the next several weeks, doctors tried to treat her disease and save her unborn child. But her condition worsened. It soon became clear that unless she had an abortion, her chance of dying was "close to 100 percent."

Three weeks later, on November 27, when the woman was on the verge of death, hospital physicians consulted St. Joseph's medical ethics board and its director, Sister Margaret Mary McBride. Recognizing that four children were about to lose their mother, McBride approved the abortion and the woman's life was saved.

The abortion at St. Joseph's soon came to the attention of Thomas J. Olmsted, bishop of the Catholic Diocese of Phoenix, who immediately excommunicated McBride and severed ties with the hospital. The seven-hundred-bed hospital was asked to remove the Blessed Sacrament from its chapel and told it could no longer celebrate Mass. "The direct killing of an unborn child is always immoral, no matter the circumstances," said Olmsted, "and it cannot be permitted in any institution that claims to be authentically Catholic."

St. Joseph's Hospital is one of six hundred Catholic hospitals in the United States; forty-five are sole providers for their communities.

DURING THE PAST FEW YEARS, books written by non-believers have become quite popular; most notably, *The God Delusion* by Richard Dawkins; *The End of Faith* by Sam Harris; and *God Is Not Great* by Christopher Hitchens. All of these books claim that religion is illogical and potentially harmful. I assumed that, as I uncovered story after story of medical neglect in the name of God, I would come to the same conclusion. But I didn't. Somewhere during the process of reading large sections of the Old and New Testament, I changed my mind, finding myself largely embracing religious teachings. Sort of like the man who went to church to find God, but found religion instead.

The Old Testament contains hundreds of *mitzvahs*, or good deeds (literally, commandments). To be a good Jew means to perform those deeds—to honor your parents, family, friends, neighbors, and strangers with acts of selflessness. The New Testament isn't much different; at its heart is the fundamental message of Jesus Christ: *But now faith, hope, and love, abide these three; but the greatest of these is love* (1 Corinthians 13:13). Sometimes this passage is interpreted as *faith, hope, and charity.* In either case, to be a good Christian means to be a loving person; to be charitable; to care about those around you, especially those who are suffering or in need. As a pediatrician, I was most affected by Matthew 25:40: *Verily, I say unto you, Inasmuch as you have done it unto one of the least of my brethren, you have done it unto me:* a passage that could be emblazoned onto the entranceway of every children's hospital in the world.

What I have learned is that to be truly religious is to be humane; to find that greater part of ourselves; something that causes us to do extraordinary acts of love and kindness; that allows us to see ourselves as part of a larger community. In the name of religion, people have counseled the addicted, ministered to the downtrodden, fed the poor, housed the homeless, helped tsunami victims, and served as beacons in the fight against slavery and for civil rights. But religion has also been used to justify some of humankind's most unconscionable acts. This book is about trying to understand why we allow that to happen; why we allow people to claim that they are acting in the name of God when they are doing no such thing.

One story summarizes the point of this book. In 2014, our infectious diseases team at The Children's Hospital of Philadelphia was asked to evaluate a little girl who suffered from bacterial meningitis. She came into the hospital with fever and seizures. Despite antibiotics, the fever continued. So did the seizures. Eventually her brain pushed down onto her brainstem, causing her to stop breathing. Now she's in a vegetative state, unlikely to see, hear, speak, or walk ever again. Her parents had chosen not to vaccinate her for religious reasons. Given that the strain of bacteria that caused her disease was preventable by a vaccine, it was an unfortunate choice. During rounds, I felt like doing something that I obviously could never do: walk into the room; put my arms around the parents; point to their comatose, helpless child; and ask, "Does this look like a religious act to you? Do you really think that God wants your child to suffer like this? Is this what religion is all about?"

THE READER WILL BE SURPRISED to learn that the hero of this book isn't science or medicine or doctors; it's religion. The journey will include understanding how organized religions can become destructive cults; exploring the psychological forces that have allowed some parents to watch their children slowly die from treatable diseases— often knowing that the diseases were treatable; examining how literal interpretations of religious scriptures have been used to justify some of our most inhumane acts; explaining why American politicians, prosecutors, and judges have been limited in their ability to protect children from harm caused by certain religious rituals—a problem caused when two Watergate co-conspirators threw a wrench into the justice system; and, perhaps most difficult of all, tackling the issue of abortion in an attempt to understand the line that separates respect for the unborn child from disregard for the pregnant woman.

ALTHOUGH MANY OF THE STORIES you are about to read are unimaginably painful and sad, one stands above the rest. It's the story of a mother who found order in chaos, humanity in alienation, and redemption in sin. The worst kind of sin.

This book will begin and end with her.

1

"THE VERY WORST THING"

"You always think you know the worst thing.
But it's never the very worst thing."

—RICHARD FORD, *CANADA*

Rita Swan was born in 1943 in Ogden, Utah, the first of six children. When she was four, her father converted to Christian Science. Soon, both her mother and father experienced Christian Science healings. The father, whose doctor had given him "pink medicine and brown medicine" for a throat condition, threw the medicine down the toilet and quickly recovered. The mother, who had been burned by lye while scrubbing floors, converted when the burn marks on her hands miraculously disappeared. All six children were raised without medical care. All survived.

Rita enthusiastically embraced the religion of her parents. "I prayed for the animals when they were sick. For the ones that recovered, we gave credit to Christian Science. One time our cat was bitten by a snake and his face swelled up. So we gave him a treatment, which is an argumentative form of prayer. It argues that the disease is unreal because God didn't make it and God is good and God is the only power. You just have to keep arguing to convince yourself that the disease is an illusion. It's an error. It's not part of God's creation. In reality you are a perfect image of God so you can't be sick and you keep formulating these arguments to yourself over and over again until the disease disappears." When the cat recovered, the family gave him a Christian Science name. They called him "The Demonstrator."

The Swan family had embraced a relatively modern religion, established only seventy years before Rita was born. It was founded by a woman who was at one time homeless, but who died a millionaire.

MARY BAKER EDDY was born on July 16, 1821, in Bow, New Hampshire, the youngest of six children. Her father, Mark Baker, was a justice of the peace and a Congregational Church deacon. Her mother, Abigail, believed Mary was a Divine Spirit sent by God.

As a child, Mary suffered a variety of illnesses. "Mary Baker's 'fits' frequently came on without the slightest warning," recalled a contemporary. "At times the attack resembled a convulsion. Mary pitched headlong on the floor, and rolled and kicked, writhing and screaming in apparent agony." Her father would hitch up the wagon, and maniacally flog the horses on the way to the doctor's office, all the time shouting, "Mary is dying!"

Eddy's illnesses persisted. Throughout adolescence she was gravely ill one minute and fine the next. One biographer described her as "an anthology of nineteenth century nervous ailments." Because Mary believed her symptoms were brought on by noise, she covered a nearby wooden bridge with sawdust. When that didn't work, she killed the frogs outside her home.

By the time she was an adult—and had gone through two marriages and given birth to a child whom she later abandoned—Eddy had experimented with a variety of treatments to cure her ailments. She had tried mesmerism (hypnosis) and special diets. She had tried homeopathy, where medicines are diluted to the point that they aren't there anymore. And she had tried hydropathy, drinking large quantities of water. But her moment of clarity came in June 1862, when she visited the Vail Hydropathic Institute in Hill, New Hampshire. It was there that Eddy heard about a man who would change her life and provide the philosophical basis for her soon-to-be-founded religious movement. His name was Phineas Parkhurst Quimby.

QUIMBY WAS THE SON of a blacksmith. As a young man, he was fascinated with electricity and magnets, believing they had curative powers. Although poorly educated and largely illiterate, he founded a healing cult that centered on hypnotism, massage therapy, and the power of suggestion. Quimby argued that if emotions can cause physical illnesses—as Freud later proved—then all illnesses could be reversed by the right kind of thinking. "Disease is a belief," he declared.

In October 1862, when she was forty-one years old, Mary Baker Eddy visited Phineas Quimby at the International Hotel in Portland, Maine. She wanted him to treat her back pain. After she was cured—and inspired by Quimby's power-of-suggestion therapy—Eddy set upon a path to cure others. Unlike Quimby, however, Eddy's healings had a theological underpinning. In February 1866, after she slipped on the icy streets of Lynn, Massachusetts, Eddy turned to the Bible for relief, reading the passage about Jesus's healing of a paralyzed man. Later, she testified, "Ever after I was in better health than I had before enjoyed." Eddy had experienced her epiphany. She would create a religion that combined Quimby's power of suggestion with the healing ministry of Jesus. Christian Science was born.

At first, Eddy's healings resembled those of the psychics, spiritualists, and mediums of her day. She held séances, claiming to see spirits of the departed. And she fell into trances, supposedly locating lost items, missing persons, and—in one inspired moment—Captain Kidd's buried treasure.

In 1875, Eddy wrote *Science and Health with a Key to the Scriptures*, the book that would become the bible of her religion. (And a book she would revise about three hundred times.) Seventeen years later, she founded the mother church of Christian Science in Boston. Eddy believed that the material world, which includes sin, illness, falsehood, poverty, war, and death, is just an illusion—as is the physical body. The only realities are God and his spiritual mirror image: man. She reasoned that because all diseases are caused by ignorance of God, the only way to treat them was to draw closer to God through prayer.

Eddy had gone one step beyond Quimby. Although Quimby believed that all diseases were the consequence of mental states, he still believed that diseases existed. Eddy, on the other hand, believed that diseases were imaginary. Whereas Quimby believed in mind over matter, Eddy didn't believe in matter. "You say a boil is painful," wrote Eddy, "but that is impossible, for matter without mind is not painful." Because boils don't exist, they don't need to be lanced.

Eddy used the term *Science* because healings could be demonstrated, and *Christian* because healings follow the ministry of Jesus. Christian Science, however, differs from Christianity in nearly every central doctrine; most importantly, whereas Christians believe that Jesus died for their sins, Christian Scientists believe that Jesus died to prove that diseases aren't real. As for the word *Science*, Christian Science doesn't incorporate any known scientific discipline. Arguably, Christian Science is neither Christian nor Science.

MARY BAKER EDDY's philosophies captivated a nation.

By 1925, more than two hundred thousand people were Christian Scientists: a growth rate that exceeded every other religion. Christian Science churches could be found in every state, and Christian Science reading rooms in most cities and towns; all luxuriously appointed, all further evidence of the religion's newfound financial prowess.

The success of Christian Science in the late 1800s and early 1900s can be explained in part by the woeful state of medicine at the time.

When Eddy was formulating her theories, medicine had little to offer apart from quinine to treat malaria, a vaccine to prevent smallpox, and ether and chloroform for general anesthesia. Treatments consisted of emetics, bloodletting, scarifications, and corrosives. Worse, therapeutic standards, physician licensing boards, and hospital accreditation committees didn't exist. Anyone could call himself a doctor, and did. Hucksterism was rampant. Ben Franklin suggested that prayer worked because it allowed people to avoid doctors, who usually did more harm than good. One anatomist said, "The only difference between a young and an old physician is that the former will kill you and the latter will let you die." But Christian Science was different; liberating. Eddy's religion put the power to heal in the hands of the people, offering control where there had been none and hope where there had been little. And, more than any other church, Eddy empowered women—providing them with jobs as spiritual healers.

Medical science, however, didn't stand still. Before Eddy died, both a vaccine to prevent rabies and a serum to treat diphtheria became available. Soon, proof that specific germs caused specific diseases led to lifesaving sanitation programs. But Mary Baker Eddy continued to ignore the scientific advances around her. "If I harbored the idea that bacteria caused disease," she said, "I should think myself in danger of catching it." By 1910, the year of Eddy's death, salvarsan, the first antibiotic, had been invented; syphilis was now a treatable disease. Two years later, phenobarbital, the first medicine to treat epilepsy, became available. Within a decade of Eddy's death, insulin was isolated; within two decades, penicillin was discovered. Medical schools now had to be licensed, and physicians had to pass qualifying exams. In the midst of all of these discoveries, however, Christian Scientists remained firmly planted in the past, refusing to embrace a wealth of medical advances; choosing instead to believe that illnesses were imaginary and that the only road to cure was prayer.

IN 1944, RITA SWAN'S FATHER was drafted into the army, causing the family to move to posts in San Antonio, Texas; St. Cloud,
Minnesota; Lawrence, Kansas; Pocatello, Idaho; and Ogden, Utah,
eventually settling in Pittsburg, Kansas, where they operated a small
farm. "We were poor," recalled Rita. "My father sold livestock and
feed supplements on commission. I grew up in a two-bedroom home
with six kids in the Flint Hills of Kansas with no running water, no
central heat, certainly no air conditioning, and no indoor plumbing.
My three brothers slept in one bed. My sister and I slept in bunk
beds in the same room. The baby slept in my parents' room."

The Swans were largely isolated in their beliefs; Rita was the
only Christian Scientist at her rural high school. "I didn't really
have friends at all," she recalled. "I just didn't fit in. They weren't
interested in me. I couldn't sing. I couldn't dance. I didn't know
any popular music. I didn't have contemporary clothes. I felt
alienated. No one would extend themselves to me. My only sat-
isfaction was getting A's. But it wasn't a class that respected intelligence. Fewer than 5 percent of our class went to college back in
those days."

When she was sixteen years old, Rita Swan graduated as the
valedictorian of her high school class. In the fall, she attended Kansas State Teachers College in Emporia, Kansas (now Emporia State
University), and quickly joined a Christian Science organization on
campus: "That's where I met my husband. I went to a Christian Science meeting and he was there on the doorstep. We began dating
and were engaged three or four months later. I was seventeen years
old. Doug was the first guy I had ever dated."

After Rita's freshman year at Kansas State Teachers College,
Doug went to Michigan State University to get a master's degree in
mathematics. Two years later, in 1963, Rita graduated from college,
married Doug, and moved to Elsah, Illinois, the home of Principia
College—the only Christian Science college in the world—where

Doug taught math. Rita taught English at Monticello College, an all-girls school ten miles down the road. "It was quite a plum, a mark of prestige," recalled Rita. "Suddenly we were living in a community that was entirely Christian Science. And they all seemed to be making it work. They never got sick that we knew of. They gave testimonies at church about their healings. And they were very happy people. They never complained. As far as we could tell, they lived up to all the ideals of Christian Science."

Doug eventually earned a PhD in mathematics from the University of Vermont, and Rita a PhD in English from Vanderbilt University. Her dissertation was on Percy Shelley and British Romantic poetry.

THEN RITA SWAN FACED the first major test of her faith.

On October 20, 1969, Rita celebrated the birth of her first child, Catherine. Soon after, Rita suffered abdominal pain and irregular vaginal bleeding. "I was petrified," she recalled. "I had lots of Christian Science treatments, and sometimes the pain would go away dramatically." Sometimes, it wouldn't go away.

In 1976, after Rita became pregnant with her second child, Matthew, the pain returned. "During my fourth month of pregnancy I suffered extreme, severe abdominal pain on my left side, really excruciating pain." Because Christian Science allows for prenatal care, Rita went to a doctor. (Mary Baker Eddy had allowed doctors to attend Christian Science births following a lawsuit involving the death of both a mother and her newborn.) "He felt this thing growing on my left side and asked me to get an ultrasound." The doctor was convinced that Rita had either an ovarian tumor or an ovarian cyst.

Rita immediately sought out a Christian Science practitioner who assured her that the mass was just an illusion: "The doctor doesn't know what he's talking about," the practitioner reassured. "It's all just speculation." After several intense sessions of Christian

Science prayer, Rita had her ultrasound. The tumor was gone. "I thought Christian Science had accomplished a miracle," said Rita. "I thought it had dissolved this growth that the doctor was feeling. I told the Christian Science practitioner and she was walking on air. We thanked God. We praised God." The doctor, now convinced that Rita was suffering from an ovarian cyst, explained that cysts can either twist and cause pain or rupture and cause massive bleeding. Either way, he predicted that Rita's ordeal wasn't over.

Six weeks after Rita delivered Matthew, the doctor felt the growth again. "I was just devastated," recalled Rita. "Because you have this Christian Science faith that this is an absolute healing straight from God. I went home and told the Christian Science practitioner and she was devastated, too. But she said that we would work it out in Christian Science." And so Rita Swan, with the help of her practitioner, prayed.

When Matthew was seven months old, the pain returned—this time, worse than ever. "I woke up in the middle of the night with vomiting and excruciating pain on my left side," she recalled. "When the baby woke up, Doug brought him in for me to nurse. But I was just physically incapable of doing it. I was in too much pain. So I called the doctor and got him out of bed on a Sunday morning and he said that I needed to come down and be examined. That the cyst had probably twisted. The decision was a struggle. I thought maybe I would just get a shot of pain medicine. That way I could nurse my baby." (Mary Baker Eddy also permitted pain medicines because she had used them for her kidney stones—prayer, apparently, not having worked as well.) The doctor refused. "'I just cannot give you a shot and send you on your way,'" he said. "So I had the emergency surgery, and the doctor said that the cyst had ruptured and that blood was coming down into the Fallopian tube, which was a genuine medical emergency."

Rita paid a price for abandoning her faith. Placed on probation, she was no longer allowed to hold meetings at the church or teach Sunday school. Rita accepted her punishment. "I thought it made sense because I felt that I couldn't be a good representative of the faith to children after I'd had the surgery. I couldn't tell them these Christian Science truths when I had violated them." "Rita couldn't teach Sunday school because she was impure," recalled Doug.

CENSURED BY THE CHURCH she loved, Rita Swan missed the harmony and glory of her faith, missed the chance to live in a more perfect world. Asked why she later chose to return to Christian Science, Swan explained, "People said that we were afraid of losing faith in front of our church members or that we wanted to fit in. But it's really just a fear of medical science, a fear of the mortal world. The only way that a Christian Scientist is going to demonstrate his salvation is to believe the spiritual truths, believe that man is just a spiritual image of God and that that's the only way to have a harmonious life. If you believe that you are a perfect mirror image of God, you don't have poverty, you don't have wars, you don't have fatigue, you don't have an inharmonious marriage, you don't have unemployment, you don't have disease, and you don't encounter mean people. The only way to have a life that's fulfilled and purposeful and harmonious is to tell yourself every day that you live in the Kingdom of God. God has made this perfect, beautiful world for you to live in, and you can control your experience by the way that you think about it. So you're very busy. Christian Science is a hard-working religion. It's many hours a day in which you have to argue with yourself. You tell yourself you're not in a traffic jam because God's ideas always move harmoniously with each other and don't come in conflict. And pretty soon the traffic jam clears up and you've had a

Christian Science demonstration. And if the traffic jam doesn't clear up right away then it's an opportunity for more spiritual growth. So you just keep working on it until you learn deeper truths. And you're grateful to have learned those truths."

Rita Swan's return to Christian Science meant that she would now once again be living in a world free of disease. "If you go to a doctor you're just going to become subservient to the doctor's thinking," she recalled. "And doctors believe that man lives in a mortal material body. So if you went to a doctor the doctor's false thinking would contaminate your thinking. I mean, golly, there'd be hundreds of diseases that you'd never even heard of that you'd become vulnerable to." "Doctors are flooding the world with diseases," wrote Mary Baker Eddy in *Science and Health*.

When Matthew Swan was fifteen months old, Rita and Doug would be tested once more. This time, they would pass the test—and their son would lose his life.

On Friday, June 17, 1977, worried that Matthew was having trouble walking, Rita Swan called Jeanne Laitner, a Christian Science practitioner, who prayed for him. The next morning Matthew developed a fever. Then, he vomited. "I'm afraid Christian Science isn't getting to the root of the problem," Swan confided to Laitner. But Laitner was unfazed. "You don't give up on the arithmetic book," she said, "just because you can't work out all the problems." According to Laitner, Matthew's fever was a manifestation of Rita's fear, her failure to fully embrace God and His majesty.

The next day, Father's Day, Rita woke up and brought Matthew into bed with her. "Good morning, Christian soldier," said Doug. But Matthew was in a daze, unresponsive to his father's playfulness. Rita called Laitner several times that day, worried that the fever had continued, unabated. Again, Laitner reassured her that Matthew's fever was imaginary.

On Monday morning, Laitner came to the Swans's house to see Matthew. "She saw me in tears," recalled Rita. "She saw a child motionless, immobile, and expressionless." Laitner stayed for fifteen minutes, declaring, "Matthew, you cannot be sick! God is your life! You live in the Kingdom of God!" That evening Matthew's fever was the highest it had ever been. He hadn't sat up, crawled, or walked for three days. Laitner visited the home again that night, reassuring the Swans that Christian Science parents often overrate their children's illnesses. "They almost always imagine the worst thing," she said. "It's a fascination with fear."

On Tuesday morning, Rita called Laitner to say that Matthew had a small fever blister in his mouth, which had started to bleed. Laitner was unconvinced. Fever blisters didn't exist. If you believed in God, believed in His power, you could ignore what you thought you saw. "If you're relying radically on God," said Laitner, "it doesn't make any difference what the evidence is."

Later that afternoon, Matthew had trouble swallowing. Again, Laitner visited the home. Matthew's fever raged on; he couldn't sit up or, according to Rita, "do the hundreds of other beautiful things he had always done." After examining Matthew, Laitner was convinced that her prayers were working. "He *is* making progress!" she insisted.

On Wednesday morning, Matthew lay quietly in his bed, rarely moving. Rita called Laitner one more time, looking for something—anything—that would tell her the tide was turning. Laitner was unfazed, again insisting that Matthew was getting better. "I suggested she could come for another house call," said Rita, "but she didn't think it was necessary. 'Now that Matthew has turned the corner,' she said, 'his progress in Christian Science will be steady and sure.'"

On Thursday morning, with Matthew struggling to eat, Rita reached a crossroads. "We decided we must either change practitioners or turn to medicine," she recalled. "We had been trying so hard to do what Jeanne wanted us to, yet our baby was still sick. I was afraid it would take too much time to 'get into' another practitioner's approach. But I was even more terrified of turning away from Christian Science and the only concept of God I had ever known." Christian Science practitioners are instructed not to pray for anyone who voluntarily accepts medical care. If the Swans took Matthew to a doctor, there would be no going back. So Rita and Doug decided to switch practitioners instead.

THE SWANS CALLED JUNE AHEARN, who had prayed for one of Matthew's fevers two months earlier. Ahearn was initially suspicious. Why would the Swans change practitioners? Were they dissatisfied with the results? Or, worse, had they considered medical treatments, something Mary Baker Eddy had referred to as *materia medica*? "I'm getting a strong message of temptation towards *materia medica*," said Ahearn, "and I want to ask you quite frankly if there has been any history in your family of resorting to modern medicine?" Ahearn warned that doctors "could do nothing for you," and that if her prayers were to work, Rita's "reliance on Christian Science had to be total."

The next morning, Friday, Matthew screamed whenever Rita touched his back or neck. Ahearn believed she knew what the problem was: Rita had never resolved a distant relationship with her father. If Matthew was to be healed, Rita had to write a conciliatory letter to him. Ahearn explained how she had once healed gallstones by getting a patient to confess resentment toward a relative. So Rita wrote the letter.

On Saturday, the Swans asked June Ahearn to come to their house and look at Matthew, instead of praying from her home. "When June had first taken the case, we had brought up the idea of a house call," recalled Rita. "She said she didn't need to see Matthew because her business was understanding him as a spiritual idea. From then on, I was afraid to show any disagreement with her attitude by asking her again. When I phoned Sunday morning, though, June offered to stop by after church. That morning, before she arrived, I lay on the floor sobbing and shouting, 'He is just a baby,' over and over."

On Sunday, around midnight, Matthew began screaming uncontrollably. By 1:15 A.M., Rita couldn't take it anymore; she called Ahearn for an urgent prayer session. Ahearn said that the problem might not be Rita's unresolved relationship with her father; but rather that she had used a different practitioner before her, a practitioner who obviously didn't know what she was doing. According to Ahearn, Jeanne Laitner's previous "mental malpractice" had made it impossible for her to heal Matthew. Rita didn't know what to do. So she grabbed *Science and Health*—the Bible of her religion—the book that contained everything any good Christian Scientist needed to know. Over and over, she read the passage, "Divine Love has always met and will always meet every human need."

But Matthew's screaming continued.

On Monday morning, the Swans had an idea: something that would enable them to take Matthew to a doctor without violating the rules of their church. Christian Scientists are required to report any contagious disease to local health authorities. This would allow doctors to visit Matthew. When Doug raised the idea to Ahearn, she dismissed it. "You're too concerned about what the community thinks," she said. Ahearn predicted "a long, hard road back to Christian Science if [the Swans] turned to medicine."

On Monday evening, Matthew lay quietly in his bed, unresponsive. "I held a strawberry before his face, telling him about it over and over," recalled Rita. "After many minutes, he began to extend his hand towards it. With excruciating effort, he coordinated his hand to the strawberry and with equally painful effort got it to his mouth and chomped on it mechanically." It would be the last bit of solid food Matthew Swan would ever eat. "Around nine that evening I was rocking Matthew in his room and trying to feed him again," recalled Rita. "His face, tilted towards mine, was distorted. His eyes would not blink. They were bugged out and bloodshot. It was just too horrible. I put him back in his crib and called Mrs. Ahearn."

Now June Ahearn was really frustrated. She had worked hard on Matthew's case, praying several times a day, yet Matthew didn't seem to be getting better. "I'm not going to be one of those practitioners who brag about working for hours over and over," she told Rita. "I've done my work on this case for the day and that's that. Now it's only been an hour and a half since you [last] called. He can't possibly be in bad shape. It's you and Doug with your fear that are holding this whole thing up!" If Matthew was to get better, the Swans were going to have to become less fearful of their son's illness.

On Tuesday morning, Matthew, too sick to scream, just moaned incoherently. The next day, in excruciating pain, he began to gnash his teeth. "Maybe he's gritting his teeth because he's planning some great achievement," suggested Ahearn. "Why don't you take a positive interpretation of the evidence?!"

Then Matthew began to have seizures. Ahearn visited the Swans to check him out, again putting a positive spin on his symptoms. "Well, hey, what a lot of progress here," she enthused. "Look how active he is. If there's movement, Divine Mind is directing it." To June Ahearn, Matthew's seizures could be a good thing.

On Thursday morning, Matthew Swan was delirious. Ahearn wondered whether he had always been somewhat delayed; maybe that's why he seemed slow to respond to her prayers. "How mentally active was Matthew before?" she asked. "The question tore my heart out," recalled Rita. "Matthew had always been such a bright, happy, robust boy. He banged on the piano so enthusiastically that his chubby bottom left the bench. He slid down the stairs on his tummy at top speed. He climbed the ladder of the highest slide all by himself. He flooded our days with the ecstasy of discovery and achievement, desire and fulfillment. Now, suddenly, he had lost recognition of everything. We didn't know how or why. But [for her to ask] how 'mentally active' he was before he got sick. I managed to control my anguish enough to say that he had always been very bright." Ahearn acknowledged that she "never knew him very well."

THEN JUNE AHEARN GAVE Rita and Doug Swan a way out—a chance to get Matthew the care he needed while still saving face with the Christian Science Church. "Maybe Matthew has a broken bone in his neck," said Ahearn. "I remember you said he fell off the bed once." (Christian Scientists are allowed to see doctors to set broken bones.) Within an hour, the Swans walked into St. John's Hospital, where the doctor ushered them into a treatment room, immediately surrounded by six nurses. After a brief exam, the doctor asked Rita how long Matthew had been unresponsive. "His voice was kind," recalled Rita. "He only wanted information. But I stared at him in shock and could not say anything. Really, Matthew had not been responding for twelve days." Swan didn't answer the pediatrician's question, saying only what June Ahearn had told her to say: Matthew needed to be checked for a broken bone.

Confident that she had followed her practitioner's instructions, Swan called Ahearn to let her know what was happening. "I didn't tell you to take him to the hospital!" shrieked Ahearn. "You could have just taken him to an X-ray clinic!" Rita returned to the treatment room only to find another pediatrician, Dr. Sharon Knepfler, asking Doug a series of rapid-fire questions. "Like the six nurses, she was purely and totally focused on saving a child's life," recalled Rita. "They were a stunning contrast to the Christian Science nurses, who had been called by a desperate mother on Monday morning and still weren't there on Thursday, and the practitioners with their accusations, excuses, and denial of Matthew's suffering."

Dr. Knepfler explained that Matthew had bacterial meningitis complicated by an abscess, a collection of pus deep within the brain. If Matthew was to have any chance of survival, the abscess needed to be drained by a neurosurgeon. Doug asked if they could get a second opinion but was told there wasn't time. The Swans consented to the surgery, later calling Ahearn to let her know where things stood. "I called June back with the news," recalled Swan. "She immediately dropped the case, as the Church orders practitioners to do." Ahearn accused the Swans of having questioned her healing powers from the beginning, no doubt interfering with her ability to cure Matthew. "This just shows your temptation to resort to *materia medica* that I have seen all along," she said. Ahearn offered to continue to pray for the Swan family, but not Matthew. "I didn't want her praying for us," recalled Swan. "But I was still afraid of her, so I hung up without commenting on her offer."

Knowing that the Swans were Christian Scientists, Dr. Knepfler arranged for a place near the operating room for a practitioner to pray. When it became increasingly obvious that no practitioner was coming, Knepfler said, "I know something else I could do for you. We have a priest who knows about all the different religions. Would you like him to be with you?" The Swans readily agreed.

Matthew's surgery didn't go as planned. Instead of finding a single, drainable abscess, Matthew's brain was riddled with abscesses, too many and too deep to drain. At this point, the only thing doctors could do was administer antibiotics and hope.

On Tuesday morning, an EEG showed that Matthew had suffered irreversible brain damage. Rita was desperate, still convinced that if she could only find the right practitioner, Christian Science prayer would save her son. But no one would take the case. Matthew was now in the care of doctors. From the standpoint of the church, he was out of its hands.

On Thursday, July 7, 1977, Matthew Swan died of a treatable illness.

MEMBERS OF RITA'S CHURCH immediately closed ranks. Children with meningitis died all the time, they argued, especially in hospitals. "Didn't the doctors tell you he had something terminal?" asked church board chairman Jean Hawkins. "Surely Matthew's death in the hospital was evidence that medical science couldn't heal him either. Six or eight children had died in a meningitis epidemic forty miles away despite the best medical treatment in the world, while Christian Science had healed a little boy in an adjacent suburb." Hawkins was proud that Christian Science practitioners had cured meningitis when doctors couldn't. Months later, Rita Swan would dig deeper into Jean Hawkins's story of the child with meningitis who had supposedly been cured by Christian Science prayer. When she found out what had really happened, she did something that no Christian Scientist had ever done before.

The day after Matthew was admitted to the hospital, Rita and Doug Swan left the Christian Science Church, believing that the unwillingness of its practitioners to pray for their son while he lay dying in a hospital was an unchristian thing to do. "We felt that if the Christian Science church wasn't going to pray for Matthew, someone should," recalled Rita. "So my husband started calling churches of other denominations. And we came upon this woman from the United Church of Christ on a crisis line. And we went to their church on Sunday and stood up in front of the whole congregation and told them our baby was dying and we wanted them to pray for him." Which they did. Embraced by congregants of the United Church of Christ—who follow Jesus's message of forgiveness and love—the Swans never looked back. They've attended church every week for the past thirty-five years.

Several years after Matthew Swan's death, one Christian Science Church official commented on his case. "There is nothing dictatorial here," said Arthur Davies. "No one can forbid you to seek medical help." Davies was right. No one forced the Swans to do what they did. So why didn't they seek medical help earlier? How were they able to ignore Matthew's suffering for so long?

2

A FRAGILE MAGIC

"Ignorance is a shield."

—DAN SIMMONS, *THE FALL OF HYPERION*

When the dust settled, Rita and Doug Swan were angry.

First, they were angry at the Christian Science Church: "When people later asked us why we didn't take Matthew to a doctor," said Doug, "we could only say that we *did* take him to a doctor. At least what from the standpoint of the Church was a doctor."

Next, they were angry at their Christian Science practitioners: "[June Ahearn] said that because I had seen a doctor for my ovarian cyst that I'd opened up Matthew to all kinds of illness," recalled Rita, "that the sins of the parents had been visited upon the child." Doug also felt that they had been misled: "When Matthew had a fever, we had no idea what was going on. We were afraid because he had fever. But they told us it was the opposite. He had fever because we were afraid. We were demoralized because we thought we had caused Matthew's illness. We were told that if we saw a doctor, we would have broken the first commandment: 'You shall have no God other than me.' Our doors weren't locked, but we were held captive to the promise that our Christian Science healers would cure Matthew."

In fact, soon after Matthew's death, the Swans were so angry at their Christian Science practitioners that they sued them for medical malpractice. Their logic was clear. Christian Science practitioners like Jeanne Laitner and June Ahern had been trained and accredited by the Church in the art of healing. When Laitner and Ahearn prayed, the Swans understood that Matthew was being treated. Furthermore, Laitner and Ahearn billed for their services. And although the Swans didn't have medical insurance while they were living in Detroit, most insurance companies—including Michigan Blue Cross and Blue Shield—reimburse Christian Science practitioners for their time. Indeed, Christian Scientists can claim prayer as a medical deduction on their income taxes. To the Swans, this sounded a lot like a healthcare system. With one exception: Christian Science practitioners can't be held accountable for bad outcomes. Or held accountable at all.

At the time of their lawsuit, the Swans planned to donate any money they received to the National Multiple Sclerosis Society. But it never got that far. The suit was dismissed before it ever went to court. The judge claimed that Christian Science healers had been practicing their religion, not providing healthcare. Norman Talbot, a legal advisor and spokesman for the Christian Science Church, who often appeared on national television, asked, "When Jesus healed, was He practicing medicine or was He practicing religion?" Jesus, however, never billed for his services or asked to be reimbursed by insurance companies. Dr. Norman Fost, an ethicist with the American Academy of Pediatrics, put the privileged position of faith healers in perspective. "The Christian Science Church is asking to practice medicine with complete immunity from prosecution," he said. "No doctor could ever ask for that."

But mostly the Swans were angry at themselves. "Matthew died because we accepted the tenets of the Christian Science Church," said Rita. "And that is our moral responsibility." "You don't get past the guilt," said Doug. The Swans have had a tough time trying to explain just how ignorant they were about the workings of the human body. "If I had known that [Matthew] had meningitis," said Rita, "if I had known that medicine had a 95 percent chance of healing him, then I would have taken him to a doctor. I'd never been to a doctor as a child. I didn't know anything. I didn't know that a fever could mean an infection. You can't begin to understand the helplessness of someone who doesn't know anything about medicine, how vulnerable we were in the face of our ignorance." Doug agreed. "Whenever a news program came on that talked about medicine or epidemics, we were told to turn off the television," he said. "Christian Science teaches that ignorance of disease is an advantage." When asked how two people with PhDs in English and mathematics could make such uninformed choices, Rita said her knowledge of Percy Shelley's poems or Doug's of mathematical equations were useless when it came to healing their son. "A PhD will not protect you against disease," said Rita. "I literally knew nothing about medicine."

Years later, Rita Swan offered another explanation for her failure to treat her son: she had been the unwitting victim of a cult. "Christian Science has all the features of a cult," she said. "We should never have allowed ourselves to be isolated like that."

When discussing modern-day religious cults, five come to mind. Two continue to fly below radar; three flamed out in firestorms so spectacular that they attracted international media attention. All, similar to Mary Baker Eddy and Christian Science, were inspired by powerful, charismatic leaders.

ONE ACTIVE RELIGIOUS CULT is the Faith Assembly Church, a vital group with followers sprinkled across the country. It was founded by Hobart Freeman. "Our children don't know what a pill tastes like," said Freeman, "or what a doctor looks like, or what a hospital smells like, or what surgery feels like." Freeman spoke in tongues, put curses on people, and insisted that tapes of his sermons be played every hour. In one sermon, titled "The Seven-Headed Serpent,"

Freeman warned, "Hospitals are infested with evil spirits that have to leave a dead body and inhabit a living one." According to Freeman, demons entered bodies through surgical incisions. At least ninety-seven members of the Faith Assembly Church have died of treatable illnesses—almost all have been babies and young children.

Perhaps no story involving Freeman's church has been more heartbreaking than that of Natali Joy Mudd. In 1980, four-year-old Natali developed a tumor near her right eye; although malignant, it could have been treated successfully with early surgery. But Natali's parents, members of a Faith Assembly church in Indiana, chose prayer instead. The tumor grew to be the size of Natali's head. After she died, police found streaks of blood along the walls in Natali's home. Blinded and unable to stand upright, she had leaned against the walls for support.

ANOTHER ACTIVE RELIGIOUS CULT is the Followers of Christ Church in Oregon City, Oregon, which was founded by Walter White. White believed that only he could interpret God's word and, therefore, only his followers would go to Heaven; everyone else would go to Hell. White didn't believe that doctors should do anything, including setting bones or delivering babies—that is God's work.

Like members of Hobart Freeman's Faith Assembly Church, White's followers have also stood by and watched their children die in unimaginable ways. The most gruesome death involved Neil Beagley, a sixteen-year-old with a bladder obstruction. At autopsy, coroners found that urine had backed up from Neil's bladder to his kidneys, eventually bursting into his abdomen then into his lungs. The pain caused by this particular series of events is inconceivable. But Neil, with the urging of his parents, Jeff and Marci, maintained his faith, refusing to see a doctor. "You either have faith that God will heal or you seek medical attention," said Marci. "It has to be one or the other." Jeff later told investigators he was proud that his son had been true to his church. "This is who we are," said Marci. "This is what we do."

The Faith Assembly Church and the Followers of Christ Church are insular groups, sequestered from their surrounding communities. Most people have never heard of them. Three other religious cults were also insular. Or at least they tried to be. Unfortunately, because of a series of headline-grabbing incidents, almost everyone has heard of them. Indeed, when people think about religious cults, these are three that they think about.

JAMES WARREN JONES was born on May 13, 1931, in Richmond, Indiana. As a young boy, Jones was drawn to a local Nazarene church and its fire-and-brimstone preacher. "I found immediate acceptance," he said, "and about as much love as I could interpret as love." When he was sixteen, Jones preached on the streets of Richmond. Seven years later, he opened his own church. Calling it the Peoples Temple of Full Gospel Church, he encouraged both African Americans and whites to join. Before long, his flock had grown to more than two thousand.

In the early 1970s, Jones moved to Redwood Valley, California, where he ministered to the poor and destitute. According to Julia Scheeres in her book *A Thousand Lives*, "Temple members put a roof over their heads and food in their mouths. They cured heroin addicts, sitting with them around the clock until their tremors and vomiting subsided. They helped single mothers pay for schoolbooks and clothes. They brought destitute seniors to doctors for checkups. They offered newcomers a place in their home, a cup of warmth, a listening ear. Jones's ministry was based on kindness. In return the new acolytes pledged him their unswerving loyalty." Jones's good works won praise from political figures such as California governor Jerry Brown, San Francisco mayor George Moscone, First Lady Rosalyn Carter, and Senator Walter Mondale.

In the spring of 1973, Jones, intoxicated with his power and popularity, began his sermon, "For some unexplained set of reasons, I happen to be selected to be God." Then he described miracles he had performed, including resurrection. "You may not believe, but I'll tell you, there was never a miracle done in the world, 'less I did it. I am God, the Messiah." From that point forward, he insisted that congregants call him Father.

Jones soon graduated from delusions of grandeur to paranoia— certain that imagined enemies were out to destroy him. Church members had to be thoroughly frisked: combs were run through scalps, babies were unwrapped, cameras and recording devices were confiscated. To escape imagined enemies, in July 1974, Jones purchased 3,800 acres in the jungle of Guyana along the Venezuelan border, calling his new utopia Jonestown. Four years later, hundreds of his congregants followed him there. But Jones's paranoia only worsened.

In 1978, Congressman Leo Ryan Jr., a Democrat from California, traveled with a film crew to investigate claims of abuse and starvation from congregants who had escaped from Jonestown. When Ryan tried to leave, Jones's guards killed him and three members of his investigative team. (Leo Ryan Jr. is the only US congressman to have been assassinated while in office.) Ryan's death set in motion the largest mass suicide in human history. On November 10, 1978, Jones asked his followers to ingest a mixture containing grape Flavor-Aide, potassium cyanide, Valium, and chloral hydrate (colloquially known as "knock-out drops"). Jones insisted that his followers drink the mixture—children first, adults next. "Poisoned parents, weeping," wrote Scheeres, "carried their poisoned daughters and sons into the muddy field, cradling them as best they could, as their children began to convulse and froth at the mouth. They watched their kids die before beginning to strain for air themselves. The odor of burnt almonds—a telltale sign of cyanide ingestion—hung in the air." When it was over, 909 people were dead; 304 were children, 131 were under the age of ten.

VERNON HOWELL WAS BORN on August 15, 1959, to a fifteen-year-old unwed mother in Houston, Texas. By the time he was twelve, Vernon had memorized much of the New Testament, especially the Book of Revelations. Howell attended Garland High School in Dallas, but dropped out after the ninth grade, eventually supporting himself as a carpenter.

In 1979, Howell was baptized as a Seventh Day Adventist, a Protestant Christian denomination founded in the 1830s that doesn't believe in smoking, drinking, or fighting in wars, choosing instead to be conscientious objectors. Two years later, Vernon joined the Branch Davidians, a splinter group of Adventists located in Mount Carmel, Texas. The seventy-seven-acre compound located near Waco had no central heating and little indoor plumbing.

In 1984, Howell cemented his place among the Branch Davidians by marrying Rachel Jones, the daughter of a church elder. Howell was twenty-four; Jones was fourteen. Six years later, Vernon Howell changed his name to David Koresh. (*Koresh* is the Hebrew word for Cyrus, the ancient Persian emperor.) Like James Jones before him, David Koresh soon believed that he, too, had been chosen to be the Anointed One, the Messiah. When he took over the leadership of the compound, he declared, "If the Bible is true, then I am Christ."

Following his apotheosis, Koresh believed that the apocalypse was near and that he and his followers would be among those chosen for eternal life. Like James Jones, David Koresh insisted that the Davidians call him Father. Also like Jones, Koresh began sleeping with members of his group, especially adolescent girls between twelve and fourteen. One was Michelle Jones, the younger sister of his legal wife, who later bore him a daughter named Serenity Sea. Koresh had at least twelve children and several wives.

In preparation for the apocalypse, Koresh armed his compound with assault rifles, submachine guns, and hand grenades, obsessed with the imminent final confrontation between good and evil. Koresh watched and rewatched movies like *Platoon*, *Full Metal Jacket*, and *Hamburger Hill*, prompting some members of his group to call him the Rambo Messiah. Koresh's actions later came to the attention of authorities, who accused him of physically and sexually abusing children and illegally stockpiling weapons, including chemicals for the manufacture of explosives. Officers of the Bureau of Alcohol, Tobacco, and Firearms (ATF) along with the Texas National Guard surrounded the Mount Carmel compound, insisting that Koresh and his group leave.

On February 28, 1993, after a tense standoff, authorities attacked. The Davidians fought back. When the dust settled, twenty ATF officers were wounded and four were killed. Authorities retreated, marking the beginning of a tense, fifty-one-day standoff. "Whereas the faithful at Mount Carmel accepted him as a teacher, a prophet, and the Lamb of God, his opponents saw him as a con man, a poseur, and a madman," wrote James Tabor and Eugene Gallagher in *Why Waco?* The situation was unresolvable.

On April 19, 1993, ATF officers advanced, shooting canisters of tear gas into the compound. A fire broke out. Nine Davidians escaped, but seventy-four burned to death; twenty-one were less than fourteen years old. Many officials believed that the fire had been set by Koresh.

IN 1972, MARSHALL APPLEWHITE founded Heaven's Gate, a UFO-based religion located in San Diego, California. On March 26, 1997, police were called to a seven-bedroom house that featured a swimming pool, a spa, and tennis courts. There they found thirty-nine men and women in advanced stages of decay. All wore black pants, black Nike shoes, black long-sleeved shirts, and purple shrouds;

and all had plastic bags over their heads that were tied around their necks. Next to each body was a suitcase that contained underwear, sweat suits, and toiletries. Investigators later found that all had ingested large quantities of phenobarbital and vodka before putting the bags over their heads, essentially dying of suffocation. It was the largest mass suicide on United States soil.

Heaven's Gate members represented a cross-section of the American public: one was the daughter of a retired federal judge; another was a mother of five with a steady job as a postal worker; a third was from a wealthy Connecticut family; and, most famously, a fourth was Thomas Nichols, the brother of the actress Nichelle Nichols, who played Lieutenant Uhuru on the original *Star Trek* series. Others were housewives, businessmen, Army veterans, and computer scientists.

Applewhite was convinced that the Hale-Bopp comet, which had last appeared more than four thousand years ago, was a sign of the apocalypse. He also believed that trailing behind the comet was a spaceship waiting to take his group to safety. In anticipation of the spaceship's arrival, every member of the group carried a passport or identification card. A few months before the suicide, the group had purchased alien-abduction insurance for $10,000.

Applewhite left behind a video explaining his group's actions. "By the time you receive this, we'll be gone—several dozens of us. We came from the Level Above Human in distant space and we have now exited the bodies that we were wearing for our earthly task to return to the world from whence we came—task completed. The distant space we refer to is what your religious literature would call the Kingdom of Heaven or the Kingdom of God."

DESPITE THE OUTLANDISH NATURE of their actions, it would be unfair to label the People's Temple, the Branch Davidians, and Heaven's Gate as cults solely on the basis of their religious beliefs.

The difference between reputable religious groups and cults such as Heaven's Gate (which combined Christian themes of the apocalypse, martyrdom, self-denial, and salvation) or the Branch Davidians (a splinter group from the Seventh Day Adventist Church) or the People's Temple (which mimicked many Pentecostal churches) isn't the nature of their beliefs but rather the men who led the believers, all of whom had descended into madness, bringing their followers down with them.

So, was Rita Swan right? Is Christian Science a religious cult?

When it comes to organized religions, it's hard to define the word *cult*. The Oxford English Dictionary defines *cult* as "a relatively small group of people having religious beliefs or practices regarded by others as strange or sinister." Surely, faith healing sects like Christian Science are a small group. Roughly 2.1 billion people in the world call themselves Christians, a third of the world's population. Fewer than 0.01 percent of those who call themselves Christian are Christian Scientists. The second part of the definition of *cult* is that the group would have to be "strange or sinister." Any group that allows children to die unnecessarily is sinister. And if these groups invoked the name of the Flying Spaghetti Monster instead of God, their children would likely be put in foster care and their adults in an institution. But because they claim to act in the name of God, public officials often turn a blind eye.

Another way to define *cult* is to consult the world's expert: Robert Jay Lifton, a psychiatrist and professor at the City College of New York. Lifton has made his life's work studying situations in which ideology crushes humanity. In his 1961 book *Thought Reform and the Psychology of Totalism*, Lifton outlines the criteria that he believes define all cults, whether religious or political. Lifton's criteria have become a working model for psychologists, sociologists, and anthropologists. According to Robert Lifton, Rita Swan was right about Christian Science.

Cults control information. "The most basic feature of the thought reform environment," writes Lifton, "is the control of human communication." Rita and Doug Swan were instructed by their church to isolate themselves from all forms of medical information. If a television or radio program described a recent epidemic, they turned it off. If a newspaper or magazine article described a disease, they ignored it. As a consequence, the Swans knew little to nothing about health. When Matthew had a fever, Rita didn't know that fever could mean infection. Indeed, she had never owned a thermometer. Such was the completeness with which she had maintained her ignorance.

Cult leaders are chosen by God. According to Lifton, cult leaders invariably portray themselves as "agents chosen by history, by God, or by some other supernatural force to carry out the 'mystical imperative,' the pursuit of which must supersede all considerations of decency or immediate human welfare." Like James Jones and David Koresh, Mary Baker Eddy claimed Divine Will to manipulate her following. She boasted that her mother's premonition of a Divine Child matched the Virgin Mary's foreknowledge of Jesus. Eddy said that when she was eight years old, she heard a voice call out her name three times, likening it to the biblical passage where Samuel had been called three times by the Lord. According to Eddy's book, after she made her reply, "her body was lifted entirely from the bed on which she lay, to a height . . . of about one foot." Also, after she recovered from a fall on the ice in Lynn, Massachusetts, Eddy compared her recovery to Jesus's rising from the dead after the third day. And she compared her wanderings, which included several cities and three husbands, with the nomadic Jesus. In 1882, after returning from a trip to Washington, DC, Eddy wrote, "This was my entry into Jerusalem. Will it be followed with the cross?" Eddy believed that because God had chosen her to lead, her ideas, as written in *Science and Health*, were not to be questioned, even if it meant standing back and watching family and friends suffer needlessly.

Cults demand purity. Lifton argued that in cults, "The experiential world is sharply divided into the pure and the impure, into the absolutely good and the absolutely evil." Worse, that cult members often believe that "anything done to anyone in the name of this purity is ultimately moral." When Rita Swan allowed surgery for an ovarian cyst, she had become impure. As a consequence, the Christian Science Church cast her out. After she returned to the Church, she regained her purity—a purity that would cost her son his life.

Cults demand confession for imagined sins. "Closely related to the demand for absolute purity is an obsession with personal confession," writes Lifton. "There is a demand that one confess to crimes one has not committed, to sinfulness that is artificially induced, in the name of a cure that is artificially imposed. Confession becomes a means of exploiting, rather than offering solace." If Rita was to return to the church she loved, she had to confess to the "sin" of having sought out medical care. Only then would she be pure in the sight of God, only then would she be able to receive healing powers that make modern medicine unnecessary.

Cult doctrines are inflexible. "While transcending ordinary concerns of logic," writes Lifton, "[the cult] makes an exaggerated claim of airtight logic, of absolute 'scientific' precision." When Mary Baker Eddy wrote *Science and Health*, she had created the Word, which required no interpretation. Indeed, Eddy refused to have others lead services because they might interpret her writings incorrectly. Services were to be readings from her book only. Eddy's use of the term *science* is ironic given that there was nothing scientific about it. No hypothesis testing; no statistical analysis of outcomes; simply an absolute dogma written by someone who claimed to know the mind of God. Frankly, given that passages in *Science and Health* are repetitive, self-contradictory, and difficult to understand, interpretations of Eddy's writings would have been helpful. For example, Eddy wrote, "The nothingness of nothing is plain; but we need to understand that error is nothing, and that its nothingness is not saved, but must be demonstrated in order to prove the somethingness of Truth."

Cults load the language. "Cult language is repetitiously centered on an all-encompassing jargon," writes Lifton, "prematurely abstract, highly categorical, relentlessly judging, and to anyone but its most devoted advocates, deadly dull: in Lionel Trilling's phrase, 'the language of nonthought.'" The mind-defying mantra of Christian Scientists is that God is perfect; God created man in His image, therefore, man is perfect; disease isn't perfect, therefore, disease doesn't exist; disease is an illusion, ignore it. Rita and Doug Swan repeated these phrases over and over—repeated them while their son progressed from high fever to seizures to lethargy to coma, and eventually to death. Day after day they stuck to Mary Baker Eddy's "language of nonthought"—stuck to it until it was far too late to save their son.

Cult doctrine trumps experience. "The underlying assumption," writes Lifton, "is that the doctrine—including its mythological elements—is ultimately more valid, true, and real than is any aspect of actual human character or human experience." To be a Christian Scientist means to believe that much of what is happening around you is unreal. Because God created a perfect world, sin, war, disease, dishonesty, plagues, tsunamis, and infidelity don't exist; they just appear to exist. The Swans, however, didn't live in a cave. They watched television, read newspapers, and constantly interacted with people who weren't Christian Scientists. They got their PhDs in major universities. Surely they had heard of people who had seen doctors and recovered. Their challenge was to deny that this had anything to do with them, deny their experience, deny their humanity—not an easy task. "Christian Science is a hard-working religion," said Rita.

Cult doctrine trumps existence. "Existence comes to depend upon creed (I believe, therefore I am) and upon submission (I obey, therefore I am)," writes Lifton, who argues that none of us is that far away from this; that at some level we all yearn for "a supernatural force that will bring solidarity to all men and eliminate the terror of death and nothingness." Like all religions, the doctrine of Christian Science offers something greater than that found in our earthly existence. According to Lifton, the line that separates cults like Christian Science from other organized religions is the degree to which people are willing to deny their humanity in the name of that doctrine.

In the United States, tens of thousands of Americans belong to more than twenty different faith healing sects—all of which could reasonably be considered cults, using Lifton's criteria. In addition to Christian Science, other groups include: The Followers of Christ Church, Faith Assembly Church, Faith Tabernacle Congregation, First-Century Gospel Church, End Time Ministries, Church of the Firstborn, The Believers Fellowship, Church of God, Church of God of the Union Assembly, First Gospel Delivery Church, Faith Temple Doctoral Church of Christ in God, Jesus Through Jon and Judy, Christ Miracle Healing Center, Northeast Kingdom Community Church, Christ Assembly, The Source, "No Name" Fellowship, The Body, One Mind Ministries, Twelve Tribes, and the Born in Zion Ministry.

MEMBERS OF FAITH HEALING cults like Christian Science aren't held at gunpoint or drugged or beaten into submission. All willingly stay and do what is instructed, even if it means watching their children die from treatable diseases. Why don't they just break away? What holds them there? If asked, most members of these cults— and frankly, most members of almost all organized religions—would probably say the same thing. Their leaders had correctly interpreted the Word of God. Therefore, they and they alone will be afforded eternal life in Heaven—a promise that causes some people to act in unimaginable ways.

3

A VENGEFUL GOD

"You see, Mr. Gittes, most people never have to face the fact that at the right time and the right place, they're capable of *anything*."

—Noah Cross, *Chinatown*

For many deeply religious people, obedience to God means a trip to Heaven, where one can live for all eternity basking in the power and the glory of the Almighty. It's an offer that's hard to resist. And when it causes people to do good deeds—such as honoring their children and their neighbors—it's a wonderful thing. Unfortunately, the promise of an eternal life can also cause people to do awful things, such as crashing planes into the World Trade Center. In a better world, we wouldn't need the promise of Heaven. We would do the right thing because it's the right thing to do—what Abraham Lincoln termed "the better angels of our nature." When Mother Teresa ministered to those living in squalor in Calcutta, she no doubt did it because she enjoyed serving God. But would she have done the same thing without promise of an afterlife—if her only reward was the smiles of those around her? One can only imagine that her answer would have been yes—the virtue of selflessness being its own reward.

Hell is also a powerful motivator.

Some of the most influential stories in the world's literature describe what can happen to someone who dares to challenge God, dares to risk eternal damnation. One involves the origin of Satan and the concept of Hell. Lucifer, the "Morning Star," the "Bearer of Light," was God's favorite angel. But when God asked Lucifer and the other angels to honor Adam—His newly designed perfect creature—Lucifer refused, arguing that Adam was a mere mortal. Angry that he had disobeyed Him, God cast Lucifer (now called Satan) down into Hell to be surrounded for all eternity by those who succumbed to his temptations.

Adam and Eve are another example of what can happen if you disobey God. Both had been granted free reign in Eden: a perfect paradise. Everything they needed was provided for them. All God asked was that they never eat from the Tree of Knowledge. Soon a serpent convinced Eve to take a bite of fruit from the forbidden tree; Eve then convinced Adam to do the same thing. The price for disobeying God was high. After losing their innocence, Adam and Eve were banished from the Garden of Eden, forced to toil and suffer on Earth.

Probably the most vivid image of God's demands for obedience is one of the first stories in the Bible. *Some time later, God tested Abraham. God said, 'Take your son, your only son, whom you love—Isaac—and go to the region of Moriah. Sacrifice him there as a burnt offering on a mountain I will show you.' Abraham bound his son Isaac and laid him on the altar, on top of the wood. Then he reached out his hand and took the knife to slay his son. But the angel of the Lord called out to him from heaven, 'Do not lay a hand on the boy,' he said. 'Now I know that you fear God, because you have not withheld from me your son, your only son.'* (Genesis 22:1–2, 9–12). Arguably, no biblical story depicts man's willingness to obey God's commands more than this one.

WHEN PEOPLE CHOOSE TO withhold lifesaving medicines from their children, the fear that holds them in place is often something unseen. Maybe it's an unspoken punishment from God, or denial of a place in Heaven, or simply the loss of a supportive community. Whatever the fear, no true believer wants to suffer the fate of the favored angel Lucifer—cast out of Heaven and condemned to serve eternity in Hell—or of Adam and Eve, cast out of the Garden of Eden and condemned to suffer on Earth. If the true believer feels it is God's will—even if it runs counter to their humanity—then they do it. They seem willing to act as Abraham acted, to sacrifice their child on a mountaintop as a show of faith. "It's hard to explain the tremendous fear that a Christian Scientist has for going to the doctor," said Rita. "[Church officials] make it very clear that the Church will desert you. We knew there would have been no going back if the doctors didn't help. Then we would have had no doctor and no God."

TODAY, MOST PEOPLE HEARING the stories of Matthew Swan or Natali Joy Mudd or Neil Beagley feel comfortable that it could never happen to them. Surely they would have responded differently to the suffering in front of them. But they shouldn't be so certain. One experiment performed in the early 1960s—perhaps the most famous social psychology experiment in history—showed how, under the right circumstances, almost anyone can do the unimaginable. The study was performed by a professor of psychology at Yale University named Stanley Milgram.

Milgram wanted to understand Hitler's willing executioners: ordinary men and women who committed extraordinarily inhumane acts. "It has been reliably established that from 1933 to 1945 millions of innocent people were systematically slaughtered on command," wrote Milgram in the first pages of his book, *Obedience to Authority*. "Gas chambers were built, death camps were guarded, daily quotas of corpses were produced with the same efficiency as the manufacture of appliances. These inhumane policies may have originated in the mind of a single person, but they could only have been carried out on a massive scale if a very large number of people obeyed orders."

Milgram wanted to understand the psychology of obedience. He had heard the oft-repeated balm that what had happened in Nazi Germany could never happen here. Americans would never submit themselves to that kind of tyranny; never follow orders that were so monstrous and inhumane. But Stanley Milgram proved that Americans were perfectly capable of doing exactly what so many citizens in Nazi Germany had done. "When you think of the long and gloomy history of man," wrote British scientist and novelist C. P. Snow, "you will find that more hideous crimes have been committed in the name of obedience than have ever been committed in the name of rebellion."

It was an unsettling experiment.

MILGRAM'S STUDY INVOLVED three players: the "experimenter," the "learner," and the "teacher." Both the experimenter and the learner were actors. The teachers were the subjects of the experiment; they didn't know that both the experimenter and the learner were merely playing a role. Milgram wanted to see what the teacher would do under extreme stress.

The experimenter was a thirty-one-year-old biologist. Dressed in a white technician's coat, he was impassive, stern, and distant. The learner was a forty-seven-year-old Irish-American accountant, described as mild-mannered and likeable. When the person under study (the "teacher") entered the room, the experimenter explained that he was investigating whether learning could be enhanced under duress. "Psychologists have developed several theories to explain how people learn," he said. "One theory is that people learn things correctly whenever they get punished for making a mistake." The task was straightforward. The teacher was asked to read a series of paired words, like *blue box*, to the learner. Then the teacher would say the word *blue* and follow it with several other words, like *sky*, *ink*, *box*, and *lamp*. The teacher would then ask the learner, who was strapped into a device that resembled an electric chair in another room, which word paired with *blue*. If the learner said *box*, then the teacher would go to the next list of words. If the learner was wrong, the subject was instructed to administer an electric shock, and to give incrementally greater shocks with each incorrect answer. "Move one lever [15 volts] higher on the shock generator each time the learner gives a wrong answer," instructed the experimenter. The teacher also had to announce the voltage level before administering the shock. If the teacher reached 450 volts, he was instructed to continue to administer the shock two more times. If the learner still didn't get the correct answer, the teacher could stop the experiment.

The shock generator looked official, consisting of 30 levers ranging from 15 to 450 volts. Above the levers were warning labels that read from left to right: "Slight Shock," "Moderate Shock," "Strong Shock," "Very Strong Shock," "Intense Shock," "Extreme Intensity Shock," and "Danger: Severe Shock." The final two levers, corresponding to 435 and 450 volts, were simply labeled "XXX." When the teacher pressed the lever, a bright red light appeared above the switch, an electric buzzer sounded, a blue light labeled "Voltage Energizer" flashed, and the dial on the voltage meter swung to the right. To convince the teacher that the learner was being shocked (which he wasn't), the teacher was attached to the machine and given a real shock of 45 volts. The teachers, however, *never* administered an actual shock during the experiment; they only thought they had.

The learner was given a series of predetermined responses to different voltage levels. He didn't express any discomfort until he was given the bogus 75 volts, at which point he gave out a little grunt.

The learner reacted similarly to 90 and 105 volts. At 120 volts, he shouted to the teacher that the shocks were becoming painful. At 135 volts, the learner gave out a loud, painful groan; and at 150 volts, the learner shouted, "Experimenter, get me out of here! I won't be in the experiment any more! I refuse to go on!" Screams and pleadings like this continued with rising intensity through 180 volts, at which time the learner cried out, "I can't stand the pain!" By 270 volts, the response was an agonized, bloodcurdling scream. From 150 volts forward, the learner pleaded to be let out of the experiment. At 300 volts, the learner shouted that he would no longer answer any questions. The experimenter would then instruct the teacher to consider no answer to be a wrong answer and to shock the learner according to the original instructions. After 330 volts, the learner said nothing; as far as the teacher knew, he could have died from a heart attack.

During the study, teachers would often look to the experimenter and ask whether they should continue. If the teacher said he or she wanted to stop, the experimenter responded with a series of four predetermined prods. Prod number 1 was, "Please continue." Prod number 2 was "The experiment requires you to continue." Prod number 3 was "It is absolutely essential that you continue." And Prod number 4 was, "You have no other choice; you must go on." If the teacher refused to obey after Prod number 4, the experiment was terminated.

Before beginning his experiment, Milgram asked psychiatrists, college students, and middle-class adults how far they thought the teachers (subjects) would go. All predicted that subjects wouldn't go beyond 135 volts, which was labeled "Strong Shock"; and all predicted that 100 percent of subjects would quit before they got to the end of the experiment. But they were wrong. Sixty-five percent of subjects went to the maximum levels, shocking the learner independent of his pleadings, his screams, and eventually his silence— shocking the victim with a voltage labeled "XXX" twice while hearing nothing from the next room. And it didn't matter whether subjects were in their 30s, 40s, or 50s; men or women; workers, students, or professionals. It didn't matter if they were housewives, nurses, engineers, medical technicians, social workers, drill press operators, welders, water inspectors, or religion teachers. Everyone, independent of gender, background, or level of education, was capable of administering what he or she thought were potentially fatal shocks to someone they didn't know simply because a man standing next to them in a white lab coat told them to do it.

Regarding the unanticipated result, Milgram wrote, "Subjects have learned from childhood that it is a fundamental breach of moral conduct to hurt another person against his will. Yet, almost half the subjects abandon this tenet in following the instructions of an authority who has no special powers to enforce his commands. It is clear from the remarks and behavior of many participants that in punishing the victim they were often acting against their own values." Yet they continued. Later, Milgram modified his experiment so that the learner was sitting right next to the subject, close enough to touch. Still, 30 percent of subjects shocked the learner up to the maximum level.

WHEN STANLEY MILGRAM published his results in 1963, many refused to believe them, arguing that his experiment didn't mimic a real-life situation; people capable of this level of inhumanity would clearly display psychological characteristics that would distinguish them from others. While Milgram was conducting his experiment, however, an event was occurring in Jerusalem that supported his conclusions: the trial of Adolf Eichmann, a notorious war criminal responsible for the systematic murder of millions of Jews.

Eichmann's trial was an international media event. Every day, people packed the courtroom, craning their necks to see what absolute evil looked like. One attendee was Hannah Arendt, a German American philosopher, political theorist, and author. Arendt later published the book, *Eichmann in Jerusalem*. Most who attended Eichmann's trial expected to see a man possessed; a sadistic, brutal, twisted man; evil incarnate. What they saw was a mild-mannered bureaucrat who had sat behind his desk and done his job. "Half a dozen psychiatrists had certified him as 'normal,'" wrote Arendt. "While another had found that his whole psychological outlook, his attitude toward his wife and children, mother and father, brothers, sisters, and friends, was 'not only normal but most desirable.'" When Eichmann was asked whether his direct role in the extermination of millions of Jews had weighed on his conscience, he "remembered perfectly well that he would have had a bad conscience only if he had not done what he had been ordered to do—to ship millions of men, women, and children to their death with great zeal and with meticulous care." (In his book *The Nazi Doctors: Medical Killing and the Psychology of Genocide*, Robert Lifton explains how the Nazis were arguably the largest and most dangerous cult in history.)

Arendt's conclusions were consistent with Milgram's. "The trouble with Eichmann was precisely that so many were like him," wrote Arendt, "and that many were neither perverted nor sadistic, that they were, and still are, terribly and terrifyingly normal. It was as though in those last minutes [of Eichmann's life] he was summing up the lesson that this long course in human wickedness had taught us—the lesson of the fearsome, word-and-thought defying banality of evil." Shortly before midnight on May 31, 1962, Adolf Eichmann was hanged, his conscience clear. He had simply been following orders.

IN THE EARLY 1960s, Stanley Milgram proved that hundreds of people could administer what they believed were potentially fatal electric shocks because they were told to do it. Yielding to authority, they had abandoned their humanity. During the Nuremberg trials, Nazi war criminals offered the same excuse: "I did what I was told."

If Stanley Milgram could get hundreds of study subjects to perform unconscionable acts simply by hiring someone to wear a white lab coat and speak in an official manner, it shouldn't be too hard to understand how people can counter their humanity if they believe it to be God's will—a God who has the power to reward their faithfulness or punish their disobedience for all eternity.

MARY BAKER EDDY's Christian Science, James Jones's People's Temple, David Koresh's Branch Davidians, Marshall Applewhite's Heaven's Gate, Walter White's Followers of Christ Church, and Hobart Freeman's Faith Assembly Church represent extremes. Reasonable people could probably never imagine joining religious cults such as these. They're simply too foreign, too otherworldly. But most people who choose religion over modern medicine aren't members of cults, aren't ignorant of medical advances, and aren't isolated from their communities. One, Larry Parker, wrote a book about it. Called *We Let Our Son Die*, it was later made into a movie. Parker's story provides another insight into the psychological forces that allow some parents to watch their children suffer in the name of God, knowing full well that they could have prevented that suffering.

4

THE FAITH HEALER
NEXT DOOR

"The beauty of religious mania is that it has the power to explain everything. Once God or Satan is accepted as the first cause of everything that happens in the mortal world, nothing is left to chance, or change. Once such incantatory phrases as 'we see now through a glass darkly' and 'mysterious are the ways He chooses His wonders to perform' are mastered, logic can be happily tossed out the window. Religious mania is one of the few infallible ways of responding to the world's vagaries, because it totally eliminates pure accident. To the true religious maniac, it's all on purpose."

—STEPHEN KING, *THE STAND*

"The Devil made me do it."

—FLIP WILSON, AMERICAN COMEDIAN

In the early 1970s, Larry and Lucky Parker lived with their four children in Barstow, California, a town of twenty thousand people located halfway between Los Angeles and Las Vegas. All the Parker children were healthy except for eleven-year-old Wesley, who had suffered from diabetes since he was six. Larry was responsible for giving him his daily insulin injections. Unlike the Swans, the Parkers

clearly understood the nature of their son's illness and the conse-
quences of not treating it.

The story of Larry and Lucky Parker, as told to Don Tanner,
can be found in the book, *We Let Our Son Die: A Parents' Search for
Truth*. As described in that book, in February 1972, after returning
from school, Wesley lay down on the couch, groggy and disoriented.
Larry was the first to recognize what was happening; Wesley's blood
sugar was dangerously low—a consequence of having received the
wrong form of insulin. The Parkers rushed him to Barstow Community Hospital, where they met Dr. Robert Chinnock. "Wes was back
to his old self within a day or so," recalled Larry. "We felt indebted
to this specialist after that, and were impressed enough to make him
Wesley's physician. We appreciated him for teaching us how to keep
Wesley's diet better balanced to minimize insulin reactions and what
to do in case of an emergency." Larry also understood what could
happen if Wesley received too little insulin. "With too little insulin," wrote Larry, "blood sugar would be high, bringing frequent uri-
nation and loss of strength. Pain in the joints, head, and stomach
would come next, followed by diabetic coma then death."

On August 22, 1973, when Larry Parker decided to stop giving
his son insulin, he should have known what could happen.

ALTHOUGH LARRY HAD BEEN told that Wesley would need insulin
injections for the rest of his life, he believed that God heals. "I had
seen it," he wrote. "Cancer, shattered bones, blasted minds, touched
by the power of God."

The Parkers were members of the First Assembly of God
Church, a traditional church led by Pastor Gary Nash. One Sunday,
Nash turned things over to Reverend Daniel Romero, an evangelist. Romero told the congregation that through prayer, he had been
healed of a painful spinal condition. As the service ended, Romero
invited "anyone who needs a miracle in their life" to step forward.

Lucky saw the moment as a chance to rid her son of a lifelong illness. The session was dramatic. Taking Wesley firmly by the shoulders, Romero asked:

"Do you believe that God loves you?"

"Yes," said Wesley, tears welling up in his eyes.

It wasn't the first time the Parkers had turned to God for help. Two years earlier, after being laid off from his technician's job at the Goldstone tracking station, Larry had enrolled in Bible College in Santa Cruz, California, hundreds of miles from Barstow. After six weeks, he dropped out, ran out of money, couldn't sell his house, and welcomed his fourth child into the world. But Parker knew that God would take care of him and his family. "I looked forward with excitement to see how He was going to provide for our needs," he wrote.

LATER THAT DAY, OVERWHELMED by his session with Reverend Romero, Wesley declared himself healed. But that evening, Larry struggled. "What if Wesley shows sugar in his urine tomorrow morning?" recalled Larry. "What should I do? What do I tell him?" "Lord, forgive me," he thought. "Wesley is healed. Your Word promises. . . ." Larry stayed up most of the night.

Larry Parker woke up at 8 o'clock the next morning. "The struggle from the previous night returned," recalled Parker. "What if Wesley's test shows he needs insulin? Give him an [insulin shot]? No. I'm going to stand on God's Word. He must honor His Word. If the test is positive, it's a lie from Satan and I'm not going to believe external signs."

That morning, Wesley went into the bathroom and tested his urine. The testing strip turned positive, indicating large amounts of sugar—clear evidence that Wesley needed insulin. Larry recalled the moment that would eventually cost his son his life: "My heart broke as he reluctantly gestured for me to give him his shot. His small face carried years of disappointment and despair in that one moment. 'Wesley, we're not going to believe that test. It's just a lie of Satan. You are healed.'" Parker then took the insulin syringe away from his son and threw it into the wastebasket.

WESLEY BEGAN TO URINATE more frequently, evidence that he was spilling massive amounts of sugar into his urine—evidence that he desperately needed insulin. Then Wesley did something he hadn't done in years: wet his bed. "Wes had wet the bed before, when his diabetes had gotten out of control," recalled Larry. "This was a sure sign that he was craving insulin. Again, doubt and confusion filled my mind. Should I continue to claim Wesley's healing when the obvious symptoms showed that he was not? Was this also a lie of Satan, intended to make me deny my son's healing?"

Larry refused to succumb to Satan's deceptions. To prove his faith, he took Wesley's entire supply of insulin to a local dump and threw it away. But Wesley continued to suffer, now with intense stomach pains. Parker watched his son stumble out of bed—weak and dehydrated—and drag himself to the bathroom where he threw up. "Dad, my stomach hurts again, and my head aches," said Wesley. "I hurt all over. Please pray for me." Larry called Lucky, who had been praying at a friend's house with members of her church. Lucky was reassuring. Within minutes, Lucky's prayer group filed in. All stood in Wesley's room, praying: "Lord, we pray for strength," they said. "Heal Wes, dear Jesus. Let the manifestations of your healing process appear even now. We command these symptoms to go and Satan to loose his hold on this boy, in Jesus's name." Wesley asked them to be quiet; his head was throbbing. The prayer group continued to pray silently in the next room.

Then Larry sought the solace of his friend Karl Kessler, "a strong Christian who knew his Bible." Larry confided, "It's so hard to watch your son suffer like that, especially when you know that if you give him insulin, he's going to stop suffering. Yet if I do that, Karl, I'd be going against what God wants." Kessler agreed to join the vigil. But Wesley only worsened, continuing to vomit, urinating frequently, and drinking water in a ferocious attempt to stave off dehydration.

Wesley started to hallucinate, asking his mother to attend to his infant brother, who Wesley believed was outside the house. Lucky interpreted this to mean that the Devil wanted her to stop praying. Seeing the battle as a war with Satan, Lucky vowed to press on. At 3:30 A.M., Wesley Parker's breathing became more labored. Things were getting worse. And Larry was at his wits' end. "Burying my face in our son's bed, [I let] out my anguish in fervent prayer. 'God, heal my son . . . in Jesus's name!'" he demanded loudly.

Not everyone bought into the Parkers's delusion. As Wesley sank deeper into the coma that would mark the end of his life, Pastor Nash and a friend, Mark Benkowski, paid him a visit. Seeing that Wesley was critically ill, Nash and Benkowski pleaded with the Parkers to take him to a hospital. "I appreciate your anxiety," Larry said, "but I'm Wesley's father, and God has given *me* the faith. I must act on it." Parker continued to pray. "Oh, God, *Your* Son suffered only three hours, Wes has suffered for days. Oh, . . . God, why do You delay?" Lucky now believed it was possible that God had a different plan. "Could it be that God wants us to be willing to let Wesley die so that he can be resurrected?" she asked, weeping. Larry later said, "You could be right, yesterday my eyes fell on Acts 4:10 where the words were underlined *whom God raised from the dead*! Maybe that's what God wants. Maybe He wants to see if we're willing to go all the way with Him. Then we'll see Wesley's healing complete."

DURING THE FINAL MOMENTS of their son's life, the Parkers huddled together to sing a hymn:

Tis so sweet to trust in Jesus
Just to take Him at His Word . . .
O for grace to trust Him more.

When they finished, the Parkers noticed that Wesley's feet were cold and gray. Their son was dying. "The more that we became aware that Wesley was dying," recalled Larry, "the thicker the atmosphere of peace became. It was a peace that passes all understanding." Larry then announced to his prayer group, "Wesley's with Jesus now, but he'll be coming back."

"AN IDEA BEGAN TO FORM in my mind," Larry wrote. "Maybe we should take Wesley to the church. What a setting for his resurrection—up near the altar, where he had been prayed for so many times for healing. Perfect!" So he called Pastor Nash and described his plan. Nash was horrified to learn Wesley had died. "Larry, you should have talked with me about this!" he shouted. "I told you to take that boy to a doctor!" Later, Pastor Nash visited Larry and told him he was all wrong and that "God's not going to bring Wesley back from the dead." "When he does," snapped Larry, "then you'll have to apologize."

WESLEY PARKER'S FUNERAL received national attention, with interview requests from northern California, Chicago, and Los Angeles, including Regis Philbin. In a room "jammed to capacity," Larry took center stage. "It says in the Gospel of John, chapter eleven, that Jesus raised Lazarus from the grave," he began. "And that's what we're here for today—to see the bodily resurrection of Wesley Parker, one of Jesus Christ's own. Just like Lazarus, he will rise." Larry asked others to join him in prayer; when they finished, he gazed at his son's casket. Nothing. "Wesley, rise up in the name of Jesus," he implored. Still nothing. "Wesley, I command you to rise in Jesus's name."

Embarrassed silence. Then a guitarist played *Tis So Sweet to Trust in Jesus*. The casket remained still. Someone shouted from the audience, "Larry, I think the Lord wants all of the children to call Wesley back to life." The Parkers's two daughters, Pam and Tricia, walked up to the casket and prayed; soon other children joined in. "Wesley, Wesley, rise Wesley!" Again, nothing. A young man stood up and said, "The ground upon which you are standing is holy ground." A hush fell over the crowd. Larry interpreted this as a sign from God. "Just like it says in Exodus," said Larry, "when Moses saw the burning bush and heard those very words, we should remove our shoes." Larry thought he might have pinpointed the problem: nonbelievers in the audience hadn't removed their shoes. So he walked up and down the aisles, carefully checking everyone's feet.

Then a young man with a beard approached Larry and asked that he be allowed to pray for Wesley alone. Larry thought perhaps the man was an angel sent by God to answer his prayers. "Yes, of course," he told the man and asked everybody to leave. The Parkers also walked out, waiting anxiously for the bearded man to emerge with good news. "The chapel doors opened suddenly, and the youth emerged slowly from the auditorium," recalled Larry. "Hope burned in our eyes, then faded as he met our gaze dejectedly, tears disappearing in his beard." There would be no resurrection today.

A reporter came up and asked, "What now, Mr. Parker? Your son did not rise." Larry countered, "It's just like Lazarus when he was raised from the grave. We'll allow Wesley to be buried; and then God will raise him up after four days. That's what's going to happen!" On August 27, with neither of his parents present, Wesley Parker was buried at the Mountain View Cemetery. Two days later, the Parkers were arrested for murder. Charges were later reduced to felony child abuse and felony manslaughter. But Larry knew the real reason for the arrests. "We were being persecuted for our faith," he said.

WHILE AWAITING TRIAL in the San Bernardino County jail, Larry encountered a deputy who asked, "You're the one who prayed for his son to be healed and then let him die?" Larry said that he was, but that his son would soon be raised from the dead. "You know, I attend a church here in San Bernardino," said the deputy. "You've caused quite a ruckus in our congregation—some people are saying you were arrested for your faith." Comforted by the deputy's apparent support, Larry said, "Now I know how Paul the Apostle felt when he was arrested." "Yeah, but Paul was put into prison for doing the Lord's work," said the deputy. "Already feeling judged and condemned," wrote Larry, "my heart sank once more." (Presumably, Larry's likening himself to the apostle Paul was a reference to Roman persecution of early Christians for threatening the social order. Larry, too, had threatened the social order, but not the one he had in mind; in this case, it was the social order that values parents who protect their children from harm, whether in the name of God or otherwise.)

To protest what he believed was religious persecution, Larry decided to fast. After turning away a few meals—and angering his jailers—he again put his fate in God's hands. Parker believed that if his next meal was unpalatable, then the Lord wanted him to continue to fast. If it was delicious, then the Lord wanted him to eat. Parker didn't have to wait long to find out. In the upper left hand corner of his metal dinner tray was a suspicious looking brown slop. Parker tasted it, uncertain of what he would find. But the concoction had a sweet, pumpkin flavor. It was delicious. So Parker ate it all. "The Lord answered my prayer," recalled Larry, "but not in the way I had expected."

Later, Pastor Nash came to the prison to tell Larry that his children had been placed in Juvenile Hall. Larry reached his boiling point. Angry at a God who would let this happen, angry at his confinement, angry at the unfairness of being at once faithful and treated badly, he shouted, "God! God! God! When will I get outta here? How are we going to get outta here?" Then he heard a strange voice. "Patience son, soon." It was a voice that Larry knew to be that of the Lord. "He had heard me!" he declared.

WHEN THEY WERE FREE on bail, the Parkers decided to return to their church; but they were no longer welcome in Barstow. "Some of the people had turned their backs on us," recalled Larry. "Others had instructed their children not to play with ours." So, the Parkers drove thirty miles to Victorville, seeking the solace of an evangelist named Dick Mills, who echoed the words of Pastor Nash. "It was wrong for you to force this upon your son," he said. Still, the Parkers refused to admit that they had done anything wrong. "But we didn't force anything upon Wesley," Larry insisted. "When his urine test showed he needed insulin, Wes prepared his injection as usual. But I told him the symptoms were just a lie from Satan, and he was healed. Wes was thrilled. But if he'd asked for the insulin during the suffering we would have given it to him immediately." Mills softened. "God, right now, is flooding me with love for you," he said. "And I feel like He wants you to know that He loves you very much. The Lord is going to bring you into new relationships, and give you new friends as the result of Wesley's death." The Parkers were relieved and grateful. "God truly did care for us," recalled Larry. "And He had the circumstances of our lives under control."

THE TRIAL OF LARRY AND LUCKY PARKER began in a San Bernardino courtroom on May 22, 1974. Pastor Nash was among the first to testify. Nash had written a letter to his church following Wesley's death, which was read to the jury. "Dear Church member, As pastor I was opposed to the methods used by those praying for the healing of Wesley Parker. I say with full assurance in my heart that it was not of God and voiced my opinion of this to Larry Parker prior to the death of Wesley. There was a witness present who also endeavored to advise Larry Parker. Our advice was rejected. I believe in the gifts of the Spirit, but God does not have to permit a small child to go through suffering and torment, die, and be resurrected." Nash was then questioned about his church's position on faith healing. "As far as the church is concerned," asked prosecutor Tom Frazier, "the acceptance or rejection by an individual of medicine is not a criteria for determining faithfulness, is it?" "No, sir," replied Nash. (Although Nash clearly distanced himself from the Parkers at trial, he wasn't immune to the notion that God could heal through the touch of a holy man. It was Nash, after all, who, according to Larry's book *We Let Our Son Die*, had invited Reverend Romero to speak at his church: an event that later influenced the Parkers to withhold Wesley's insulin.)

Cindy Wilson, a friend of the Parkers who had prayed for Wesley in his final hours, also testified. Cindy described her beliefs. "If you believe in God," she said, "you have to believe in the Devil, too. He has power, too. He can deceive you." Frazier asked, "Do you think it is possible for the Devil to deceive people from time to time?" "Yes," replied Cindy. Frazier followed up: "And that some things that people might believe are from God may actually be from the Devil?" "Yes," said Cindy. As other witnesses testified, Larry kept coming back to Cindy's testimony. "My thoughts were haunted by her statement," he recalled. "Were Lucky and I deceived?" Had it been Satan, and not their faith in God, that had caused Larry and Lucky to do what they had done?

By the time Larry Parker took the stand, he had come to believe that Satan had deceived him and that his attempts to make God prove Himself were misguided. When he was asked whether, in retrospect, he should have done anything differently, he replied, "Yes. We should have administered the insulin to eliminate the suffering while we continued to trust God for Wesley's healing."

The trial lasted thirteen weeks. When it was over, the jury found Larry and Lucky Parker guilty on all counts. But instead of receiving what could have been a twenty-five-year prison sentence, Judge J. Steven Williams sentenced the Parkers to five years of probation. Prosecutor Frazier was beside himself. "Your Honor," he said, "the defendants in this case acted in such a manner that their conduct resulted in the death of their son. [Wesley] died at the hands of the parents and there are additional children resident in this home. The probation report indicates that numerous people interviewed as a result of the investigation feel that Mr. and Mrs. Parker are good parents. Yet I cannot help but ponder—what is a good parent? One that would permit such a thing to come to pass?" Judge Williams responded by saying, "They most certainly are guilty. The jury that prayerfully deliberated this case arrived at that judgment. However, I am sure that the defendants feel that they have the Lord's forgiveness—and without presuming on His mercy—I hope that such is the case." The Parkers wouldn't spend another day in jail. Under the terms of their probation, they had to maintain employment, report to their probation officer once a month, receive eighty hours of psychological counseling, serve four hundred hours in a work-sentence program, violate no laws, neither leave the state nor change residence or employment without permission, report any illness of a family member, and refrain from advising, suggesting, or implying to anyone that they should not seek or follow medical advice. If they agreed, they would be allowed to raise their remaining children.

The Parkers willingly accepted the terms of their probation and were grateful that they had been the recipients of many gifts from God. "During the trial," recalled Larry, "we were without definite income. Nevertheless, the Lord had been supplying our needs—checks accompanied letters of encouragement; groceries were provided; a Christian garage mechanic who had repaired our car's brakes had even given us a month to pay. When our air-cooling system broke, a plumber fixed it without charge. God had taken what Satan intended for harm and turned it around for our good."

After the Parkers had completed four of their five years of probation, they returned to court to ask that the length of their probation be reduced. Judge Williams decided to reduce their convictions from a felony to a misdemeanor. "Lucky and I were innocent of all charges," Parker later wrote. "We were free. Free from the bondage of guilt and shame that had tormented us through our ordeal. Free from the stigma of felony convictions. Free to grow into a new abundant life of Christian maturity and balance."

WHILE IT IS EASY TO EXPLAIN how Wesley Parker died, it is much harder to explain why he died. Unlike the Swans, the Parkers were medically sophisticated, having administered Wesley's insulin for years. And they weren't members of a faith healing group. Indeed, Pastor Nash had pleaded with them to see a doctor. So it's hard to use religion alone to explain their choices. Rather, it might be more useful to focus on the Parkers as individuals, not as members of a group. Was there something in the Parkers's psychological makeup that explains how they could have done what they did?

To address the forces that motivated the Parkers would require more than simply reading Larry Parker's book, which was written seven years after Wesley's death. But it might be of value to use the Parkers's story to examine hypothetically the factors at work in a case as dramatic as this one.

To determine whether someone has a psychological disorder, psychiatrists turn to the Diagnostic and Statistical Manual of Mental Disorders (DSM). According to the criteria set forth in this manual, theoretically the Parkers could fall into one of three categories. The first two are personality disorders; the third is more extreme.

One possibility is that the Parkers suffered from Dependent Personality Disorder, described in part as "a pervasive and excessive need to be taken care of that leads to submissive and clinging behavior."

Both Larry and Lucky Parker were the products of broken homes. To handle his feelings of isolation and rejection, Larry sought out an Assemblies of God church when he was only six years old. Lucky, too, was isolated as a child—raised by her aunt and uncle after her mother had suffered a nervous breakdown. One could argue that, to the Parkers, God was their surrogate parent. As a consequence, they often relied on God to tell them what to do and when to do it. When Larry lost his job, he prayed. He also prayed when he couldn't sell his house or afford his children's food and clothing. And when he was in prison, separated from his wife and children, when he most needed to take control of his life, he asked God to send him a sign, something that would tell him what to do. Although many people pray when faced with misfortune, the Parkers's passivity—as described in Larry's book—seemed far more extreme.

Larry Parker's unrealistic dependence on God culminated in the death of his son. One would like to believe that if Wesley had been standing in the middle of a street with a car approaching, Larry would have pulled him out of the way—not prayed for the car to stop. Yet in a comparable situation, when Wesley faced a deadly but treatable illness, the Parkers chose prayer instead of insulin. Like frightened children, they sang *Tis So Sweet to Trust in Jesus* while their son lay dying. Years later, in another book, Larry would reassess the events that led to his son's death.

ANOTHER POSSIBILITY is Narcissistic Personality Disorder, defined by the DSM as "a pervasive pattern of grandiosity, in fantasy or behavior, a need for admiration, and a lack of empathy."

When Pastor Nash pleaded with the Parkers to take Wesley to the hospital, Larry said, "God had given *me* the faith." After Larry was arrested, he likened himself to Paul the Apostle. When Larry asked God to set him free from prison, God talked to him. When Larry wondered whether he should fast, God sent him a delicious helping of sweet potatoes. All of these behaviors might reasonably be considered manifestations of a narcissistic personality.

In the end, Larry Parker believed that God would cure his son's diabetes and later bring him back to life because he had asked Him to do it. To Larry, God was like the CEO of his own personal "make-a-wish foundation," ready to reward his faithfulness whenever asked; like many believers in faith healing, he had presumed to know the mind of God. Although too late for his son, Parker later recognized the flaw in this presumption.

IN A MORE RATIONAL WORLD, someone like Larry Parker might not be labeled with something as gentle as a personality disorder. In my view, he would be considered psychotic, meaning "possessing a distorted or nonexistent sense of reality." Unfortunately, for people with strongly held religious beliefs, it's often difficult to know where to draw the line between faith and delusion. For example, Larry had believed that his son's physical deterioration was a trick played on him by Satan. Larry reasoned that Wesley wasn't really sick; he was well. The Devil was testing Larry's faith by making it *look* like Wesley was sick. It's hard to label this kind of thinking as anything other than delusional. But many Americans believe that the Devil roams the earth and works his deceptions. So, in some ways, Larry Parker represents a cultural norm. The same can be said for Larry's belief that Wesley's funeral service was being held on holy ground, causing him to ask everyone to remove their shoes, or for his belief that God had sent an angel—in the form of a bearded man—to help with the resurrection. Many religions claim holy ground, and many people believe in angels and demons. Again, Larry Parker is far from alone.

Larry harbored two beliefs, however, that even the most devout Christian would likely consider delusional. First, he believed he could cure his son's diabetes with prayer. As Larry knew, children develop diabetes when their pancreas stops making insulin. He also likely knew—as explained by Dr. Chinnock—that children who stop making insulin don't spontaneously start making it. But Larry believed that faith was strong enough to do something that had never been done before—cure diabetes.

Again, however, if Larry Parker's actions are to be considered psychotic, we would have to similarly label all those who participated in his delusion, including Lucky, her prayer group, and everyone who showed up at the funeral service hoping to see a resurrection. Even Lucky's lawyer, Leroy Simmons, reassured her during the trial that he, too, believed in faith healing. And we would also have to label as psychotic fifty thousand Christian Scientists and tens of thousands of Americans who comprise the twenty or so other sects that embrace faith healing.

Furthermore, if we are going to call anyone who believes in resurrections *psychotic*, remember that Oral Roberts, a popular evangelist, claims to have performed them. Although these resurrections surely never happened, no one rushed to put him in an institution after he made the claims. Indeed, many members of Roberts's congregation believed him. This is not to say that one couldn't reasonably label as psychotic all those who share the Parkers's deluded beliefs in faith healing and resurrection. It's just that you get to a point where so many people share a certain belief that calling them all delusional becomes harder to do.

IN THE END, LARRY PARKER didn't have the support of some of his Christian friends because he had violated Christianity's fundamental message: *But now faith, hope, love, abide these three; but the greatest of these is love* (1 Corinthians 13:13). Not faith, love.

THIRTY YEARS AFTER the death of Wesley Parker, Larry wrote another book: *No Spin Faith: Rejecting Religious Spin Doctors*, a passionate exposé about the faith healers whom he believed had misled him and his son—faith healers who had been under the influence of Satan. "This book is meant to encourage those who have tried to claim a healing and failed," he wrote. "Don't berate yourself with the thought, If only I had had enough faith or If only I had believed strongly enough my [child] would have been healed. Those erroneous thoughts bring condemnation, which is not from the Lord. . . . It comes from our adversary the devil. He laughs at us for being taken in by leaders whom he has used to spin God's Word into something it is not."

Parker's mission is to teach others not to make the same mistake that he had made. "To use scripture to demand whatever you want from God is not faith," he wrote. "It is presumptuous to claim that God will do something when He has not yet told you He will do it. . . . I succumbed to this teaching and withheld insulin from my diabetic eleven-year-old son. To our shock and grief, Wesley died. I believe the Lord has now assigned me to alert the body of Christ to the deception of this teaching."

One faith healer targeted in Parker's book was Kenneth Copeland, whose ministry was at the heart of a massive measles outbreak six years later.

5

THE LITERAL AND THE DAMNED

"We are punished by our sins, not for them."

—ELBERT HUBBARD,
AMERICAN AUTHOR AND PHILOSOPHER

Perhaps the simplest explanation for religiously motivated medical neglect is that some people choose to interpret the Bible literally and without question. The logic of faith healing is simple: if the Bible says it, then it must be so. Before the Parkers withheld insulin from their son, they read Mark 11:24: *Whatever things you desire, when you pray, believe that you receive them, and you shall have them.* They read Matthew 18:19: *Anything that they shall ask, it shall be done for them by my Father who is in Heaven.* And they read John 5:7: *If you abide in me, and my words abide in you, you shall ask what you will, and it shall be done unto you.* Larry Parker remembered asking himself, "Aren't we Christians living for the Lord in His perfect will? Yes. Then why shouldn't these words of Jesus be applied to us?" "Who," asked Larry Parker, "is a greater healer than God?"

Faith-healing parents often reject medical advances because they're a product of man, not God—a position that is not only illogical, but inconsistent. Let's assume the following. One: God created man in His image. Two: that image includes a brain. Three: the human brain is responsible for scientific and medical advances.

The New Testament was written about eighteen hundred years before antibiotics, clotting factors, and insulin were discovered; that's why these therapies are never mentioned. Other scientific advances also aren't mentioned. For example, centuries passed before refrigeration and pasteurization were found to reduce contamination of food and beverages; or before high-powered lenses allowed people to see distant stars or low-powered ones to read books; or before it was understood that water—if it was to be safe—had to be separated from sewage. And although all of these inventions were a product of man, the Swans, Parkers, Mudds, and Beagleys embraced them. They didn't pray for toilets or refrigerators or safe water or eyeglasses; they paid for them. But when it came time to save their children's lives, they demurred. "I do not feel obliged to believe that the same God who has endowed us with sense, reason, and intellect," wrote Galileo, "has intended us to forgo their use."

THE PROBLEM WITH literally interpreting the Bible also extends to Jehovah's Witnesses, who point in part to Acts 15:29 to explain why they reject blood transfusions, even in the most dire circumstances: *You are to abstain from food sacrificed to idols, from blood and from the meat of strangled animals.* Acts was written around AD 60. The first successful blood transfusion was in the early 1800s. One can reasonably assume that when Acts was written, people hadn't imagined that one person's blood could save the life of another. Indeed, at the time of Jesus, physicians—largely influenced by the teachings of Hippocrates—*removed* blood from patients to treat diseases. (This practice, called bloodletting, survived well into the nineteenth century.)

Despite their abhorrence of blood transfusions, Jehovah's Witnesses aren't faith healers. When they're sick, they go to the doctor. But when it comes to blood transfusions, they share one thing in common with all faith healers: a remarkable capacity to live with their own inconsistencies. Although Jehovah's Witnesses don't accept transfusions of *whole blood*, they do accept transfusions of *fractioned blood*. The logic here is obscure. Acts was written well before doctors knew that blood could be divided into a solid fraction, containing red blood cells, and a soluble fraction containing albumin, clotting factors, and nutrients. It's hard to claim Divine Will as a reason to embrace one blood component over another.

LITERAL INTERPRETATIONS of the Bible also extend to a rather surprising modern-day practice: exorcism.

In 2003, Tamara Tolefree paid a visit to Pat Cooper, the mother of an eight-year-old boy named Terrance Cottrell Jr., whose autism had become increasingly more difficult to handle. Tolefree suggested that Pat should bring Terrance to her church, the Faith Temple Church of Apostolic Faith.

Founded in 1977 and located in a Milwaukee strip mall between a pizzeria and a dry cleaning store, the Faith Temple Church contained a small stage, ten pews, and a half dozen ceiling fans. David Hemphill was the church pastor; his brother, Ray, was the church evangelist. Ray was also the church exorcist. "He has the gift to cast out devils," David explained.

The church held two services a week, both on Sundays. It wasn't long before Pat Cooper was a regular, convinced she had finally found a place that could help her son. It didn't work out that way. When Terrance's behavior worsened, the social worker assigned to his case threatened to remove him from her care. Isolated, scared, and with no support from Terrance's father, Pat was at her wits' end. But Tamara had a solution. "Terrance wasn't only suffering from autism," she said, "but also from demons in his soul."

At first, churchgoers offered special prayers for Terrance. When that didn't work, they asked Ray Hemphill to perform an exorcism. So, on the evening of August 22, 2003, Hemphill placed Terrance on the floor, wrapped him in a sheet, pinned down his arms and legs, and put his knee on the boy's chest. Hemphill leaned over and screamed, "In the name of Jesus, Devil get out!" Because children with autism are uncomfortable with physical contact— and because no child likes to be suffocated—Terrance fought to get away. Two hours later, drenched in sweat, Ray Hemphill stood up to go to the restroom. When he left, several church members walked over to Terrance, curious to see if the exorcism had worked. What they found was that he had urinated on himself, that his lips and face had turned blue, and that he wasn't breathing. One congregant called 9-1-1, but it was too late. The coroner reported that Terrance had died from "mechanical asphyxiation due to external chest compression."

Milwaukee County's district attorney charged Ray Hemphill with felony child abuse—a crime punishable by up to ten years in prison and a $25,000 fine. It wasn't the first time the Faith Temple Church had been in trouble with the law. In 1998, a twelve-year-old girl claimed to have been beaten with a stick during a church service. When the police and district attorney investigated the case, David Hemphill argued that the beating wasn't severe and that the congregation was merely doing what the Bible teaches.

In July 2004, in a trial witnessed by millions of Americans on *Court TV*, Ray and David Hemphill faced their accusers. One notable exchange occurred when prosecutor Mark Williams suggested to David that his church had taken religious healing to a dangerous extreme. Hemphill objected.

> HEMPHILL: My church is going to do exactly what the word of God tells us to do.
> WILLIAMS: So, you're saying God is giving you the power to take away. . . .
> HEMPHILL: I say He has the power! If I lay down on someone and he passes away—God took him. I didn't!

WILLIAMS: [Your brother] did it to Terrance, didn't he? Your brother did it!
HEMPHILL: No, he didn't!

On July 9, after deliberating for four hours, the jury found Ray Hemphill guilty of felony child abuse. One month later, Milwaukee County Circuit Court Judge Jean DiMotto delivered a sentence that was without precedent in the annals of American jurisprudence.

To UNDERSTAND DiMOTTO's verdict, one first needs to understand the history of exorcism, a ritual practiced by virtually every major religion.

In Judaism, exorcism is mentioned in the Talmud. To drive out the evil spirit, or *dybbuk*, a rabbi recites Psalm 91 three times and then blows the *shofar* (ram's horn). In 2012, Jewish exorcisms were popularized in the movie *The Possession*, which starred Kyra Sedgwick. Influenced by the 1914 play *The Dybbuk*, *The Possession* tells the story of Em, an eleven-year-old girl who is possessed by the spirit of a sinner seeking refuge from avenging angels. Unknown to Em or her parents, the spirit was contained in a strange box picked up at a yard sale. The box contained a lock of hair, a tooth, a bird's skeleton, an ancient ring, and unusual carvings. (All of which should have been clues that this was a box to avoid.) Soon after, Em stabs her father with a fork, fingers crawl up the back of her throat, and giant moths invade her bedroom. The family is eventually directed to an old Hasidic rabbi in Brooklyn who removes the evil spirit. *The Possession* was promoted with the question, "Thought your daughter's odd behavior was just another preteen phase? There may be an alternate explanation: the *dybbuk* is back."

Like *The Possession*, Christian exorcisms have also been popularized in movies. In 1949, doctors and psychiatrists were unable to explain the strange behavior of a teenager named Robbie Mannheim.

The boy's pastor referred him to an exorcist, Reverend Edward Hughes. Years later, William Peter Blatty wrote a book about it. Titled *The Exorcist*, the book was later made into a movie, which starred Ellen Burstyn, Max Von Sydow, and Linda Blair, and which featured the shocking image of a young girl vomiting and screaming profanities while turning her head a full 360 degrees. *Entertainment Weekly* called *The Exorcist* "the scariest movie ever made."

But when it comes to exorcisms, no group has been more enthusiastic than the Roman Catholic Church. Although exorcisms had largely fallen out of favor by the eighteenth century, recently they've made a comeback. The revival started in 1972 when Pope Paul VI declared that Satan was part of everyday life and must be defeated. "Sin, on its part, affords a dark, aggressive evildoer, the Devil, an opportunity to act in us and in our world," he said. "Anyone who disputes the existence of this reality places himself outside biblical and Church teachings." Many Americans embrace this concept; recent polls found that 40 percent believe that "people on this earth are sometimes possessed by the devil" and 70 percent believe that "angels and demons are active in the world." In June 2009, a mother in Georgia was charged with child cruelty and false imprisonment for an exorcism that involved handcuffing her teenage son to a chair while denying him food and water for three days. The judge dismissed the case saying, "I'm going to have a hard time [getting] anybody in Gwinnett County, Georgia, to say that Satan doesn't exist."

Worldwide, hundreds of exorcists practice their craft; Italy alone boasts about four hundred official exorcists. There's even an International Association of Exorcists, which holds biannual meetings in Rome and publishes a quarterly newsletter in which practitioners share tricks of the trade.

In 2005, in response to a growing demand for exorcists in the United States, the Regina Apostolorum, a pontifical academy in Rome, held an eight-week course in Baltimore to train more exorcists; sixty-six priests and fifty-six bishops showed up. Clerics were instructed on the four telltale signs of demonic possession: speaking languages that the possessed had never learned; knowing something that the possessed could not possibly have known; having strength beyond the possessed person's physical makeup; and displaying a violent aversion to God, the Virgin Mary, the cross, or other images of the Catholic faith. (Terrance Cottrell Jr. fit into none of these categories.) "What they're trying to do in restoring exorcisms," said Dr. Scott Appleby, a professor of American Catholic history at the University of Notre Dame, "is to strengthen and enhance what seems to be lost in the Church, which is the sense that the Church is not like any other institution; it is supernatural. It's a strategy for saying: 'We are not the Federal Reserve, and we are not the World Council of Churches. We deal with angels and demons.'" During the past few decades, the Catholic Church has appointed more than a dozen priests to perform exorcisms in the United States.

As Ray Hemphill demonstrated, however, exorcisms can be quite dangerous. In 1976, West Germany's Bishop Josef Stangl granted permission to two priests to exorcise a twenty-three-year-old woman named Anneliese Michel, who had suffered from depression, seizures, and hallucinations. The priests determined that the spirits of Lucifer, Adolf Hitler, Judas Iscariot, and Emperor Nero had inhabited Annaliese. For ten months, she was subjected to sixty-seven exorcisms, ending in her death. At autopsy, having suffered beating and starvation, she weighed only sixty-nine pounds. Her parents and the two priests who performed the exorcisms were convicted of negligent homicide; all received suspended sentences. In 2005, Anneliese's story inspired the movie *The Exorcism of Emily Rose*. (A documentary titled *The Exorcism of Anneliese Michel* contains the original audiotapes from the exorcisms.) Following Anneliese's death, the Catholic Church in Germany required exorcism permits.

Most Germans now have to travel to Switzerland or Poland for their spirit removals.

Anneliese Michel and Terrance Cottrell Jr. aren't the only people to have died during exorcisms. In 1997, a Korean American woman was stomped to death in Glendale, California. That same year, a five-year-old girl in the Bronx died after being forced to swallow a mixture of ammonia and vinegar, followed by having her mouth taped shut. In 1998, a mother in Sayville, New York, convinced that her seventeen-year-old daughter was possessed, suffocated her. In 2001, a Korean exorcist strangled a thirty-seven-year-old woman to death in New Zealand. And in 2014, a woman stabbed and killed her two young children during an exorcism in Germantown, Maryland.

On August 20, 2004, Judge Jean DiMotto sentenced Ray Hemphill to thirty months in prison for the death of Terrance Cottrell Jr. and ordered him to pay $1,224.75 in restitution. DiMotto also barred Hemphill from performing exorcisms *until he had received more formal training in the art*. In other words, the problem wasn't that Ray Hemphill had performed an exorcism; it was that he needed to learn a safer way to do it.

Fatal conflicts between modern medicine and biblical interpretations aren't limited to the New Testament.

In Genesis 17:10–11, God made a deal with Abraham, the father of the Jewish people: *Every male child among you shall be circumcised. And you shall circumcise the flesh of your foreskin, and it shall be a token of a covenant between Me and you.* Of the 613 *mitzvahs* (commandments or good deeds) mentioned in the Torah, circumcision—a sacred covenant between God and every Jewish male—is second only to *Be fruitful and multiply.* (Genesis 1:28) This practice, which is at least five thousand years old, has several health benefits. Circumcised men are less likely to be infected with human immunodeficiency virus (the cause of AIDS) and human papillomavirus (a common cause of anal, genital, cervical, and head and neck cancers). They're also less likely to suffer urinary tract infections. For these reasons, the American Academy of Pediatrics and the World Health Organization recommend circumcision. About one-third of the world's male population is circumcised.

The ritual, however, has a dark side.

On September 12, 2012, Sharon Otterman, a reporter for the *New York Times*, watched Romi Cohen perform a circumcision. "The *mohel* [person who performs a ritual circumcision] lifted the infant's clothing to expose his tiny penis. With a rapid flick of a sharp, two-sided scalpel, the *mohel* sliced off the foreskin and held it between his fingers. Then he took a sip of red wine from a cup and bent his head. He placed his lips below the cut around the base of the baby's penis for a split second creating suction, then let the wine spill from his mouth out over the wound." In other words, to remove blood from the circumcision site, Cohen didn't use sterile gauze; he used his mouth. The ritual, called *metzitzah b'peh* (sucking with the mouth), dates back to the Babylonian Talmud, a fifth-century text that states "the [*metzitzah*] is performed for the sake of the infant's safety. And if a mohel does not perform the suction [of the wound], this is deemed dangerous and he is to be dismissed." Although the Talmud doesn't mention how suction should be performed, the method is implied in the *Shulkhan Arukh*—the most authoritative code of Jewish law—written in the 1500s. One section, the "Yoreh Deah," states that following circumcision, "We spit blood into the earth."

The ritual of *metzitzah* was practiced throughout the Middle Ages. By the nineteenth century, however, it had fallen out of favor. Two reasons. First, Ignaz Semmelweis had established the basic principles of hygiene. Doctors now knew that the mouth contained germs that were potentially dangerous and that could be spread from one person to another. Second, *metzitzah* had caused tuberculosis and syphilis in more than seventy babies. As a consequence, Rabbi Moses Schreiber, a leading rabbinical authority, declared that blood from a circumcision should be cleaned using a sterile instrument such as a pipette; this ruling was quickly adopted by most rabbinical authorities.

But not all.

IN NOVEMBER 2004, New York City's Department of Health received a report about twin boys from Brooklyn who had each suffered a herpes simplex virus (HSV) infection. Two different types of HSV infect people: HSV-1 and HSV-2. Typically, HSV-1 is spread from the mouth, and HSV-2 is spread from the genitals. To determine how the twins had contracted the infection, health department workers went to the hospital where they had been born. They found that the twins had been delivered by Caesarian section and, as is traditional, had been circumcised when they were eight days old. One week later, they each developed blisters on their genitals, abdomen, and back. HSV-1 was isolated from both babies; one survived, the other didn't. Continuing to gather clues, investigators found that their mothers had never had herpes and that their placentas didn't show any evidence of the infection. Babies usually contract herpes *before* they're born (following premature rupture of the membranes in a woman who has genital herpes), *while* they're being born (when the child passes through a birth canal infected with herpes), or *after* they're born (when they're kissed by family members or friends who don't realize they have herpes virus in their mouths). Because the mothers weren't infected, investigators concluded that the babies must have contracted the infection *after* they had been born. So they evaluated the fourteen hospital workers who had cared for the babies. None of them had herpes. Then the investigators were alerted to another infant, this one from Staten Island, who had been infected with herpes the year before. The Staten Island baby provided the clue they needed to solve the case. All three babies had been circumcised by the same *mohel*, Rabbi Yitzchok Fischer, who had used his mouth to clean the circumcision wounds.

Eight years later, on June 8, 2012, the problem of herpes among Jewish babies received national attention when researchers from the CDC were dispatched to New York City to investigate another herpes outbreak among infants. This time it wasn't two babies who'd been infected; it was eleven. Two of the eleven had died, and two others had suffered permanent brain damage. All of the children had been circumcised by *mohels* who had used their mouths to suck off the blood. And all of the cases occurred in a zip code that contained the largest population of Orthodox and ultra-Orthodox Jews, the most fundamentalist observers of the religion. CDC investigators concluded their report with an insight into the obvious: "Circumcision is a surgical procedure that involves cutting intact skin; sterile technique should be used to minimize infection risk."

After the CDC issued its report, the mayor of New York City, Michael Bloomberg, took action. "There is probably nobody in public life who fights harder for the separation of church and state than I do," he said, "but I just wanted to remind everyone that religious liberty does not extend to injuring others or putting children at risk." New York City health officials estimated that *metzitzah* was performed on about 3,600 babies in their city every year. Armed with incontrovertible evidence that *metzitzah* was commonly practiced and potentially harmful, city legislators could have chosen to outlaw it. But they didn't. Preferring a more lenient approach, they asked only that *mohels* who used their mouths to suck blood from an infant's penis provide an educational pamphlet to parents describing the risk of acquiring herpes; *mohels* who refused to comply would be sent a warning letter and fined up to $2,000. The New York City law was the first time in United States history that the government had tried to regulate a Jewish ritual.

Arguing for the right to practice their religion freely, some *mohels* fought back. "The mayor is the mayor of New York City," said Romi Cohen, "but we have a mayor. He's the mayor of the universe. We're going to follow His instructions." Cohen, who was 83, said that he would go to jail rather than comply with the law. Others weighed in. "The Orthodox Jewish community will continue to practice what has been practiced for over five thousand years," said Rabbi David Niederman of the United Jewish Organization in Brooklyn. "We do not change. And we will not change." Some Orthodox Jewish parents were also unfazed by the risk. Isaac Mortob said he still wanted *metzitzah* performed on his first-born son. "I don't want a 99 percent job," he said. "I want a 100 percent job. I want [my son] to be fully Jewish." In the end, more than two hundred ultra-Orthodox rabbis issued a statement accusing the health department of spreading "lies and misinformation." Ordering their adherents not to comply with the city's regulation, they wrote, "It is forbidden according to the Torah to participate in the evil plans of the New York City health department in any form." On October 11, 2012, a group of rabbis sued the health department, claiming that the regulation was "in violation of their rights to freedom of speech and freedom of religious exercise."

As the conflict escalated, public health experts weighed in. "It's certainly not something any of us recommend in the modern infection-control era," said Dr. William Schaffner, chief of preventive medicine at Vanderbilt University. "This is a ritual that has now met modern science. It was never a good idea. The ancients were simply wrong about this." In response to the *mohels'* contention that they had sterilized their mouths with Listerine or wine before sucking the penis, Dr. Jay Varma, New York City's deputy commissioner for disease control, said, "There is no safe way to perform oral suction on an open wound in a newborn."

In the end, the most vocal support for the health department's position came from members of the Jewish community—most of whom were embarrassed and horrified that such an ancient, dangerous practice had survived. Rabbi Moshe Tendler, professor of Talmudic Law and Bioethics at Yeshiva University, called *metzitzah* "primitive nonsense." "The ritual has nothing to do with religion," he said. Rabbi Gerald Skolnik, president of the Rabbinical Assembly, an international association of Conservative rabbis, said the procedure was "inconsistent with the Jewish tradition's pre-eminent concern with human life and health." Even in Israel, the practice has been forbidden; in 2002, the Chief Rabbinate declared that blood from a circumcision should be removed with a sterile pipette.

Like faith healers and Jehovah's Witnesses—who often ignore some scientific advances while embracing others—*mohels* who stubbornly hold on to the ancient practice of *metzitzah* are equally inconsistent. Ancient Jewish writings describe many practices that have long since been abandoned. For example, the Mishnah, an oral history of Jewish ideas and practices, states that the open wound of a circumcision should be sprinkled with cumin. No one does this. And verses 32, 35, and 36 in Numbers 15 state, *And while the children of Israel were in the wilderness, they found a man who gathered sticks upon the Sabbath day. . . . And the Lord said unto Moses, 'The man shall be surely put to death; all the congregation shall stone him with stones outside the camp.' And all the congregation brought him outside the camp, and stoned him with stones, and he died; as the Lord commanded Moses*. Despite this biblical edict, all observant Jews refrain from killing people who ignore the Sabbath.

Indeed, *metzitzah* is a clear and direct violation of Jewish law. Whereas the government in Western cultures has a limited ability to force people to undergo any therapy that is against their wishes, such is not the case in Jewish law. In Judaism, people don't own their bodies. They're on loan, in a manner of speaking, from God. This is why followers are not allowed to get tattoos (Leviticus 21:5) or commit suicide. In a Jewish theocracy, one could theoretically force people to get lifesaving surgeries against their will. For Jews, the life and health of children are paramount. Which is why the choice of a few ultra-Orthodox Jewish sects to put children in harm's way in the name of their faith is particularly troubling.

In January 2013, a federal judge ruled against the rabbis' attempt to block New York City's directive warning parents about the possibility of herpes infections following *metzitzah*. Three months later, on April 5, 2013, two more infants were infected with herpes; in January 2014, another case was reported. In none of these instances had the parents been warned of the danger.

PARENTHETICALLY, IN DECEMBER 2013, I was asked to speak to a group of twenty pediatricians in northern New Jersey—home to one of the largest Orthodox Jewish communities in the world. I talked about vaccines. When the talk was over, several Orthodox Jewish physicians came up to the podium. Their questions showed a deep understanding of the science of vaccines and vaccine-preventable diseases. It was impressive. When they were finished, I asked how many babies in their care had been subjected to the *metzitzah* ritual. Many, they said. Then I asked how they could conscience such a procedure, knowing the potential for harm. One of the younger physicians was the first to answer. "All medical procedures have side effects," he said.

His answer took me aback. The choice to use one's mouth to clean off blood following a circumcision isn't a medical procedure. It's a religious ritual. If it were a medical procedure—and therefore required to be performed as safely as possible—blood would be removed using sterile gauze.

This interchange provided yet another insight into how people can allow religion to trump reason. When Rita and Doug Swan chose prayer instead of antibiotics for their son's meningitis, they didn't know what meningitis was; Christian Science had surrounded them with a shield of ignorance. The physician who defended the *metzitzah* ritual, on the other hand, knew that *mohels* could transmit herpes by sucking a baby's penis; knew that herpes could cause permanent brain damage and death in babies; knew that the problem wasn't just theoretical—two babies from his city had recently been hospitalized with herpes caused by *metzitzah*; and knew that the infection was completely preventable. Still, when faced with two conflicting ideologies—an Orthodox Jewish upbringing and a scientific and medical training—the doctor yielded to his religious beliefs, choosing a weak rationalization that "all medical procedures have side effects." Such is the power of religious belief.

6

DIALOGUE OF THE DEAF

"It is poverty to decide that a child must die
so that you may live as you wish."

—MOTHER TERESA

"No woman can call herself free
who does not control her own body."

—MARGARET SANGER,
AMERICAN BIRTH CONTROL ACTIVIST

When it comes to harm caused by the literal interpretation of religious texts, one issue stands above all others. An issue that undermines friendships, decides political elections, and serves as a litmus test for appointments to the Supreme Court. An issue whose rhetoric is so strident, so mean-spirited, and so unyielding that it's been labeled "the dialogue of the deaf." Abortion.

Several citations from the Bible are used to support the position that a human is a human from the moment of conception. For example, *Before I formed you in the womb, I knew you* (Jeremiah 1:4); *Your own hands shaped me, molded me* (Job 10:8); and *You fashioned me in my mother's womb* (Psalms 139:13). The most cited passage, however, is Luke 1:39–42, which refers to a meeting between Mary and Elizabeth. Mary had been pregnant with Jesus for a few days and

Elizabeth had been pregnant with John the Baptist for six months: *When Elizabeth heard Mary's greeting, the baby leaped in her womb, and Elizabeth was filled with the Holy Spirit. In a loud voice she exclaimed, 'Blessed are you among women, and blessed is the child you will bear!'*

According to the passage in Luke, Jesus was recognized as the Savior only a few days after He had been conceived. To pro-life advocates, no passage shows how destructive the taking of a life can be more than this one. However, like a number of Biblical passages, the story in Luke requires a certain suspension of disbelief. Virgin birth aside, when John the Baptist leapt for joy after sensing Jesus in Mary's womb, he was doing something that modern medicine still can't do: detect a pregnancy a few days after conception. At this point, Mary wouldn't have had any symptoms of pregnancy such as morning sickness, bloating, or an enlarging uterus. And no ultrasound in the world is sensitive enough to detect a fertilized egg. Also, because the placenta hadn't formed, human chorionic gonadotropin hadn't been released—so pregnancy tests would still be negative. Yet John the Baptist, a six-month-old fetus lacking the kinds of neurotransmitters and synapses that would have enabled one brain cell to communicate with another—allowing for emotions such as joy—leaped for joy for the unborn Jesus. The fact that modern medicine can't explain this Biblical story is, however, irrelevant. All religions require belief in a world beyond the observable laws of nature. Fair enough. So let's assume the story is accurate as written.

Much of the controversy surrounding abortion has centered on the question of when life begins. Does it begin when the heart starts to beat (around three weeks)? Or when the face starts to develop (around six weeks)? Or when the brain begins to form (around three months)? Or when the fetus starts to move (around four months)? Or when brain cells communicate with each other (around seven months)? It's an unanswerable question.

One issue about the developing fetus, however, *is* answerable. A fertilized egg, which contains a full complement of human genetic material, has the potential to become a long-lived, productive, caring human being—a fact that is undeniable. Judith Woods, a correspondent for the British newspaper *The Telegraph*, wrote, "Once you have seen four cells under a microscope in an *in vitro* fertilization laboratory and by some miracle witnessed them become an embryo, then a fetus, a baby, a little girl, it is utterly impossible not to believe that life begins at the moment sperm and egg fuse." So the relevant question isn't *When does life begin?* but rather *Should a fertilized egg be accorded the same rights as an independently functioning human being?* In the eyes of the Catholic Church, the answer to the latter question is yes. The Church does not distinguish a potential life from a life. And if one equates a potential life with an actual life, then abortion is wrong. It's a moral absolute—an understandable, logical, and consistent moral absolute.

The Church has stood firm on this issue for two thousand years. The Teaching of the Twelve Apostles, which dates back to AD 40–60, states, *You shall not kill by abortion the fruit of the womb*. In the third century, Tertullian, an early Christian author, wrote, "It makes little difference whether one destroys a life already born or does away with it in its nascent stage. The one who will be a man is already one." Centuries later, Pope John Paul II called abortion a "culture of death," and Archbishop Charles Chaput called it "murder without equivocation." In 1965, Vatican Council II condemned abortion as "an intrinsically evil act" and "an abominable crime." From the standpoint of the Church, it doesn't matter how or why conception occurred; unborn children are innocent, and aborting them is wrong.

To support the position that abortion is wrong in the absolute, however, the Church has had to live with several impractical outcomes. Every year, about 50 million abortions are performed throughout the world. If the Church's teachings were followed by everyone, fifty million more children could be born, many to unwed mothers who can't afford a child or aren't emotionally ready or don't want to bring a baby into a dysfunctional or abusive home. Because foster services are woefully inadequate, many of these children would fall through the cracks, unwanted and unloved. Furthermore, the Church doesn't seem to be particularly interested in preventing unwanted pregnancies. By failing to support sex education and birth control, it tacitly encourages unwanted pregnancies. But in defense of the Church's logic, the fact that a pregnancy is impractical or unaffordable or inconvenient isn't an excuse to end it. If you believe that a fertilized egg is a human being, then abortion is murder.

In any case, independent of one's position on the issue, abortion is an uncomfortable word. "The most striking thing about abortion is that it's ugly," writes Brian Scarnecchia, an associate professor at the Ave Maria School of Law in Naples, Florida. "There is blood, gore, and pain. In the years since abortion has been legal it has never been able to shake off the look, the smell, the sound, or the feel of the back alley from which it sprang. It is telling that for so noble a calling—that of defending the fundamental rights of women—no one wishes to be known as an 'abortionist.' There are no 'Abortionist of the Year' awards. To call a person or thing 'an abortion' is still to call it grotesque, a monstrosity."

There are moments, however, when outlawing the absolute evil of abortion becomes an absolute evil in itself.

ON NOVEMBER 3, 2009, a twenty-seven-year-old mother of four entered St. Joseph's Medical Center, a Roman Catholic hospital in Phoenix, Arizona. The woman, whose name was never released to the press, was eleven weeks pregnant and gravely ill, suffering from a disorder that caused the right side of her heart to fail. The problem had been exacerbated by her pregnancy. For the next several weeks, doctors tried unsuccessfully to treat her disease. But her condition worsened. It soon became clear that without an abortion, both the mother and her unborn child would die.

Three weeks later, on November 27, when the woman was on the verge of death, hospital physicians consulted St. Joseph's medical ethics board. The board's director, Sister Margaret Mary McBride, was the highest-ranking member of the Sisters of Mercy, an order that had founded St. Joseph's Hospital at the turn of the twentieth century. For thirty-six years, McBride had dedicated herself to healing the sick; she was experienced, savvy, and beloved. But McBride had never been in this situation before—a no-win situation. If she agreed to the abortion, she would be violating a fundamental principle of her faith. If she didn't, the woman would surely die. Recognizing that four children were about to lose their mother, McBride approved the abortion, and the woman's heart failure resolved.

The abortion at St. Joseph's Hospital came to the attention of Thomas J. Olmsted, bishop of the Catholic Diocese of Phoenix, who immediately excommunicated McBride. "The Catholic Church will continue to defend life and proclaim the evil of abortion without compromise," said Olmsted, "and must act to correct even her own members if they fail in this duty." No punishment meted out by the Church is more severe than excommunication. An excommunicated person cannot participate in the Holy Eucharist (receiving the blood and body of Christ during communion); is forbidden from holding employment in the parish; cannot participate in public worship; and is denied a Catholic burial. In short, to be excommunicated is to be exiled from Catholic society.

Despite pressure from Bishop Olmsted, the administrators of St. Joseph's Hospital didn't back down. "If we are presented with a situation in which a pregnancy threatens a woman's life, our first priority is to save both patients," said Linda Hunt, St. Joseph's president. "If that is not possible, we will always save the life we can save, and that is what we did in this case. Morally, ethically, and legally, we simply cannot stand by and let someone die whose life we might be able to save." The parent organization of St. Joseph's Hospital, Catholic Healthcare West, also supported Sister McBride. A letter written by board chairwoman Sister Judith Carle and president and CEO Lloyd Dean, stated, "If there had been a way to save the pregnancy and still prevent the death of the mother, we would have done it. We are convinced there was not." To the doctors and administrators at St. Joseph's Hospital, the choice had been clear; they could either save one life or no lives. So they saved one.

On Tuesday, December 21, 2010, Bishop Olmsted announced that the Diocese was severing ties with the hospital because it had provided care that was inconsistent with "authentic Catholic moral teaching." The seven-hundred-bed hospital was asked to remove the Blessed Sacrament from its chapel and told it could no longer celebrate Mass. "I am gravely concerned by the fact that an abortion was performed several months ago in a Catholic hospital in this diocese," said Olmsted. "I am further concerned by the hospital's statement that the termination of a human life was necessary to treat the mother's underlying medical condition. An unborn child is not a disease."

Although Olmsted implied that the Catholic Church never permits abortions, this isn't exactly the case. The most common cause of death in the first trimester is something called ectopic pregnancy. This occurs when the fetus, instead of growing in the uterus, grows in the Fallopian tubes. Untreated, the fetus eventually bursts through the Fallopian tube, causing massive bleeding and the likely death of both the mother and the fetus. In this circumstance, the Church allows the removal of the Fallopian tube, saving the mother's life and causing the death of the fetus. Similarly, if a mother has uterine cancer and requires a hysterectomy to save her life, then the procedure is permitted. Indeed, if a woman has any type of cancer that requires radiation or chemotherapy, she is permitted to save her life at the expense of her unborn child. And if a woman requires general anesthesia for surgery, the surgery is permitted even if the anesthetic would kill the fetus. All of these situations are viewed by the Catholic Church as different from the case involving Sister McBride because in none of these instances is the unborn child *directly* aborted. The abortion is indirect. In the case involving McBride, the sole purpose of the procedure was to abort the fetus. Given that the removal of an impregnated Fallopian tube or an impregnated cancerous uterus is performed to save the mother's life, the logic here is somewhat obscure.

Furthermore, while church officials claim that the life of the fetus and mother are equivalent, their actions speak otherwise. In the eyes of the Church, the fetus is an innocent; the mother isn't. No story has made the Church's preference for the unborn clearer than that of Gianna Beretta Molla, a thirty-nine-year-old pregnant woman who suffered from uterine cancer. In April 1962, rather than remove her uterus to save her life, Gianna chose to take her pregnancy to term. "If it is a question of choosing between me and the child," she said, "do not have the least hesitation. I demand that you choose the child. Save it!" Gianna gave birth to a healthy girl and died several days later. Her ultimate sacrifice led to her beatification. "Gianna Beretta Molla knew how to give her life in sacrifice so that the being which she carried in her womb could live," said Pope John Paul II. "She was aware of what awaited her, but she did not flinch before the sacrifice, thus confirming the heroic nature of her virtues. We wish to pay homage to all brave mothers who devote themselves unreservedly to their families and who are then ready to make all sacrifices. We thank you, heroic mothers, for your invincible love!"

According to the Catholic Church, the twenty-seven-year-old mother of four in Phoenix who had chosen her own life above that of her unborn fetus had acted selfishly.

ALTHOUGH SISTER MARY MCBRIDE worked in a Catholic hospital, and although her Catholic upbringing taught her that abortion was a sin worthy of excommunication, she opted to save a life rather than letting both mother and fetus die. It doesn't always work out that way.

Savita Halappanavar was thirty-one years old when she entered the University Hospital in Galway, Ireland. Born in India and trained as a dentist, Savita had followed her husband, Praveen, to Ireland, where he worked as an engineer for Boston Scientific.

In October 2012, Savita's parents spent a few weeks visiting their daughter. That's when they found out she was pregnant. "She was very excited and she said she really wanted a daughter," recalled her father. "She had a great love for the child." Praveen remembered, "She had huge expectations. She had told her friends how she wanted her baby shower to be, to bring gifts that were pink in color. She was very confident it would be a girl. She'd even thought about the name—Prasa—a combination of Praveen and Savita."

On the evening of October 20, Savita shared the news of her pregnancy with a small group of friends. That night, her back throbbing, she was unable to sleep. The next morning, she went to the University Hospital, where she was told not to worry. The baby was safe. Go home. A few hours later, the Halappanavars were in the hospital's emergency room. Large amounts of fluid were now leaking from Savita's cervix. And she was only seventeen weeks pregnant. Clearly, she was having a miscarriage. Distraught, and in a great deal of pain, Savita asked the consultant physician to induce an abortion. But she was told to let the miscarriage occur naturally. The consultant estimated that, given how much fluid was leaking from the amniotic sac, the miscarriage should be finished by the end of the day.

Late into the following night, October 21, Savita still hadn't miscarried. And her fetus's heartbeat, while weak, was still detectable. "Savita was really in agony," recalled Praveen. "She was very upset, but she accepted she was losing the baby. When the consultant came on ward rounds on Monday morning, Savita asked if they could not save the baby, could they induce [an abortion] to end the pregnancy? The consultant said, 'As long as there is a fetal heartbeat, we can't do anything.' Again on Tuesday morning, the consultant said it was the law, that this is a Catholic country. I said, 'We are not Catholics. We are Hindus. Please do the abortion immediately because her life is in danger.' The consultant said she was sorry then walked away. Savita was terribly worried and was in great pain. You would think that for humanity's sake they would have carried out an abortion. But they said there was nothing they could do. That evening, she developed shakes and shivering and she was vomiting. She went to use the toilet and she collapsed. A doctor took blood and started her on antibiotics."

At this point, Savita had been leaking amniotic fluid for three days. The fetus's heartbeat was getting weaker and weaker; it wasn't going to survive. Worse, Savita was now suffering from a serious bacterial infection that had started in her uterus and spread to her bloodstream—the dead and dying contents surrounding the fetus having served as a rich environment for bacteria to grow. To successfully treat bacterial infections, doctors must do two things: (1) give intravenous antibiotics to kill the bacteria, and (2) control the source of the infection. For example, if someone has an abscess in the liver, doctors give antibiotics *and* drain the abscess. Without drainage, the abscess can't be treated. That's because the center of the abscess doesn't have a blood supply, so antibiotics can't get in. The same was true for Savita's infection. Her uterus now contained a dying fetus and placenta, in which bacteria were growing. Without removing the contents of her uterus—by performing an abortion—antibiotics might not be enough to save her life.

On Tuesday, October 23, four days into her miscarriage and one day into her infection, doctors still refused to perform an abortion.

"The next morning I said she was so sick and asked again that they just end it," recalled Praveen. "But they said they couldn't. They said they were shifting her to intensive care. Her heart and pulse were low; her temperature was high. She was sedated and critical, but stable."

On Wednesday, October 24, when the fetal heartbeat was no longer detectable, the infected fetal contents were removed. But it was too late. "She stayed stable on Friday," said Praveen, "but by 7 pm on Saturday (October 27), they said her heart, kidneys and liver weren't functioning. She was critically ill. That night, we lost her."

Two days later, Dr. Grace Callagy performed an autopsy. Savita had died from multiple organ failure caused by the bacterium *Escherichia coli*: a common cause of genital and urinary tract infections. The doctors had appropriately given antibiotics. But by failing to remove the contents of Savita's uterus, they might have precipitated her death.

On November 3, Praveen Halappanavar took his wife back to India for cremation and a funeral. More than a thousand friends and family members showed up. "She was open-hearted and made us laugh," recalled Savita's father. "She always kept us happy. She was a kind and thoughtful girl." Said Praveen, "She was the youngest in the family and the dearest." But most of the talk that day centered on Savita's unnecessary death. Everyone said the same thing: if Savita had remained in India, where abortions are legal, she would still be alive. "There are six to seven doctors in the family—her uncle, her brother, they're all doctors—and they couldn't believe it," said Praveen. "They said it was a matter of a half-an-hour job. They couldn't believe it had happened in the twenty-first century in a country like Ireland." "In an attempt to save a four-month-old fetus they killed my thirty-one-year-old daughter," said Savita's mother. "How is that fair, you tell me? How many more cases will there be? We are Hindus, not Christians." An editorial in the *Times of India* stated, "The ban on abortion ended up taking a life that need not have been lost. How does this square with viewing the ban as 'pro-life'?"

On November 14, 2012, more than two weeks after her death, the *Irish Times* reported the story of Savita Halappanavar. Within hours of publication, two thousand people marched in Dublin to protest Ireland's abortion laws. Three days later, twelve thousand people lined the streets; one carried a sign that read, "Savita had a heartbeat, too!"

On November 19, the Catholic bishops of Ireland released a statement: "The Church believes in the equal and inalienable right to life of a mother and her unborn child and has never taught that one takes precedent over the other." Every year, more than four thousand Irish women get abortions by crossing the border to England, where they have been legal since 1967. (Prior to 1992, Irish women could be criminally prosecuted for doing this.) Unfortunately, because she was too sick to travel, Savita didn't have that option.

ONE YEAR LATER, in response to Savita Halappanavar's death, Ireland's prime minister, Edna Kenny, introduced a bill to make abortion legal if the mother's life is in danger. At the time, Ireland had the toughest anti-abortion laws in Europe. Under an 1861 law, abortions in Ireland are punishable by life in prison. Despite Halappanavar's death, Irish bishops were unrelenting, claiming the bill "represents a dramatic and morally unacceptable change to Irish law."

On May 20, 2013, Edna Kenny was the commencement speaker at Boston College, a Jesuit institution. Boston cardinal Sean O'Malley refused to attend the event.

On January 1, 2014, Edna Kenny's Protection of Life During Pregnancy Act became law.

THE PLIGHT OF PREGNANT WOMEN whose lives are in danger doesn't end with stories like that of Savita Halappanavar.

On March 4, 2009, two doctors performed an abortion of fifteen-week-old twins in the town of Recife, Brazil, a busy metropolis the size of Philadelphia. The event angered Cardoso Sobrinho, the archbishop of Recife, who immediately excommunicated the doctors. But he didn't excommunicate the mother, even though she was Catholic. That's because he couldn't. The Church doesn't allow excommunications of people younger than eighteen; and she was only nine, the victim of repeated rape by her stepfather since she was six. The girl's mother and the doctors felt it was dangerous for an eighty-pound nine-year-old to take twins to term and deliver them.

In Brazil, abortions are illegal except in cases of rape, incest, or when the mother's life is in danger. In this situation, all three applied. Although the abortion was legal in the eyes of the state, it was murder in the eyes of the Catholic Church. "The law of God is higher than any human laws," said Archbishop Sobrinho. "When a human law—that is, a law enacted by human legislators—is against the law of God, that law has no value. The good aim of saving her life cannot justify the killing of two other lives. They took the lives of innocents."

Although Archbishop Sobrinho had excommunicated the doctors as well as the girl's mother, he didn't excommunicate the stepfather, who had been raping the pregnant girl and her older sister for years. The stepfather was spared because he, too, disapproved of the abortion. "He was with us totally," said Sobrinho. "I had him at my house for the whole day. He did not accept the abortion."

Then, in the person of Archbishop Salvatore Fisichella—president of the Vatican's Pontifical Academy for Life—the Church blinked. On March 15, Fisichella issued a statement critical of Sobrinho's decision. In the Vatican newspaper *L'Osservatore Romano*, he wrote, "In the first place, [the girl] should have been defended, hugged, and held tenderly to help her feel that we are all on her side. Before thinking about excommunication, it was necessary and urgent to protect the innocent life [of the girl] and bring her back to the level of humanity of which we men of the church should be expert witnesses and teachers. Unfortunately, this is not what happened and it has impacted the credibility of our teaching, which appears in the eyes of many as insensitive, incomprehensible, and devoid of mercy." Later, Archbishop Fisichella spoke to the girl. "We are on your side," he told her. "We feel your suffering and we would like to do everything that would help you restore your dignity and [provide] the love that you will still need." While reiterating that abortion was an "intrinsically evil act," Fisichella suggested that it might have been the lesser evil.

Then Fisichella said the words that sent shock waves through religious communities throughout the world. "It is true that the girl carried within her innocent lives like her own, through the fruit of violence, and they have been done away with," he said. "However, this is not enough to pass a judgment that weighs as a condemnation." In other words, the Church should demonstrate the love and understanding that was at the heart of Christ's ministry. It was the nine-year-old girl, in addition to her unborn fetuses, who deserved the Church's mercy. Fisichella had demonstrated compassion for a child whose pregnancy would scar her for life—a child whose violent impregnation would likely define her. Or, in the words of George O'Brien, author of *The Church and Abortion: A Catholic Dissent*, precipitate "the final destruction of the spirit."

THE REACTION OF ARCHBISHOP FISICHELLA to the abortion in Recife parallels events portrayed in the 2013 movie *Philomena*, which was based on a true story.

Philomena Lee lived in Tipperary, Ireland. When she was eighteen years old, she became pregnant. Because she wasn't married—and because sex before marriage is a sin in the eyes of the Catholic Church—Philomena was sent to the Sean Ross Abbey in Roscrea, where she delivered her baby. For the next few years, the nuns at the abbey allowed Philomena to visit her son, Anthony, for one hour a day, but no more. When Anthony was about four years old, he was sold to an American couple against Philomena's will. She would never see him again.

The movie picks up the story when Philomena is in her late 60s, desperate to find out what had become of the child who had been taken from her. She teams with a journalist named Martin Sixsmith. Philomena is a devout Catholic; Sixsmith, an atheist. Eventually they discover what had happened to Philomena's son. Renamed Michael Hess, he had become a lawyer, served as a chief counsel for both Ronald Reagan and George H. W. Bush, and died of AIDS as a consequence of his gay lifestyle. Most painfully, Philomena discovers that for several years, while she had been trying to find him, he had gone back to the abbey trying to find her. But the nuns at Sean Ross had lied to both of them—telling Michael that his mother had abandoned him and Philomena that they knew nothing of her son's whereabouts (even though he was buried in the abbey's graveyard).

The essence of the movie centers on one dramatic scene, when Philomena faces the nun who had misdirected both her and her son. Seething, the nun explains that she had lied about Michael's whereabouts because Philomena, by having sex out of wedlock, had sinned against God. The nun, on the other hand, had embraced her faith, choosing a life of celibacy. Sixsmith exploded, asking how anyone could act so callously, especially someone who had cloaked herself in religious garb? "If Jesus were here today," said Sixsmith, "he would knock you right out of that wheelchair." But Philomena remained calm. "I forgive you," she said to the nun. Sixsmith stared at Philomena, angry that she had been so quick to forgive. "Just like that," he said. "That easy." "You think that was easy?" said Philomena.

The Catholic Church didn't like *Philomena*, especially the way that the nuns at Sean Ross were portrayed. "Another hateful and boring attack on Catholics," wrote Kyle Smith in the *New York Post*. But *Philomena* was very much a pro-Catholic statement. Because despite how egregiously she had been treated, Philomena Lee had never lost sight of one of the pillars of her religion: forgiveness, even in a situation that screamed for retaliation.

ARCHBISHOP FISICHELLA had refused to let narrow interpretations by other religious authorities trump his humanity. Following his statements, Catholic leaders wondered whether the Church had softened its position on abortion. They didn't have to wait long to find out. On July 11, 2009, a senior Vatican official reiterated the Church's position for anyone who thought it might have been wavering. "We have laws," he wrote. "We have a discipline. We have a doctrine of faith. This is not just a theory. And you can't start back-pedaling just because the real-life situation carries a certain human weight."

7

DO UNTO OTHERS

Do unto others as you would have others do unto you.

—Matthew 7:12

In 1997, two-year-old Michael Heilman was playing in the back-yard when his mother heard him scream. She ran out to find he had stepped on a piece of glass, his right foot bleeding. Michael's father, Dean, immediately cleaned the wound and wrapped his son's foot in a towel. But the bleeding didn't stop. So Dean rewrapped the wound in gauze surrounded by a disposable diaper. Again, the bandage quickly soaked with blood. That night Michael couldn't sleep, crying and vomiting. The next morning, the bandage was again rewrapped using a heavier fabric—but the bleeding continued. Then, instead of calling a doctor, the Heilmans called Charles Reinert—pastor of the Faith Tabernacle Congregation—and asked him to pray for their son. Later, when asked why she had chosen prayer instead of medical attention, Susan Heilman said, "When you're sick, you pray and ask the Lord to help heal you."

The cut continued to bleed, now for more than twelve hours. Michael spiraled downward. He became progressively more listless, occasionally crying out in pain. After bleeding for more than nineteen hours, Michael died in his mother's arms. An autopsy showed he had lost more than half his total blood volume. Michael Heilman had hemophilia, a disease that can be treated with blood-clotting proteins; and a problem that should have been obvious to the Heilmans, as their son had suffered frequent and severe bruising throughout his young life. Dr. Catherine Manno, a hemophilia specialist at The Children's Hospital of Philadelphia, said she had never seen a child die from a cut.

When Susan and Dean Heilman chose not to treat Michael's hemophilia, they made a choice for their son and their son only. This isn't always the case. People with certain religious beliefs can also make decisions for those who don't share their beliefs. The story that shows just how devastating such decisions can be also involved Reverend Reinert and his Faith Tabernacle Congregation. As a consequence, in the early 1990s, the city of Philadelphia was in a panic.

THURSDAY, APRIL 20, 1989

After returning from a trip to Spain, a teenager with a blotchy rash attends an R.E.M. concert at the Spectrum in Philadelphia. Within weeks, several other teenagers become sick. Measles has entered the city.

MONDAY, MAY 21, 1990

An article titled "No Measley Problem" appears in the *Philadelphia Inquirer*. The article warns that outbreaks of measles are sweeping across the country. From the comical title, readers assume that measles is probably no big deal—a childhood rite of passage. But measles can kill. And when it kills, preschool children are the ones most likely to die. Typically, they die from pneumonia (when the virus infects the lungs), or encephalitis (when the virus infects the brain), or dehydration (when the virus causes high fever, diarrhea, severe water loss, and shock). Because measles is caused by a virus, antibiotics don't treat it; only preventing the disease by vaccination can make a difference.

Before a vaccine was invented in 1963, measles infected three to four million Americans every year, hospitalizing forty-eight thousand and killing five hundred; almost all were infected by the time they were fifteen years old. Following widespread use of the vaccine, measles started to disappear. In 1978, only about twenty-seven thousand cases were reported. Encouraged, public health officials thought it was possible to eliminate the disease. So, in the late 1970s, with a goal to rid the United States of measles by October 1, 1982, they launched the Measles Elimination Program. The program was largely successful; in 1983, only about fifteen hundred cases were reported.

In the late 1980s, however, measles started to come back.

SATURDAY, JUNE 2, 1990

A couple of weeks after "No Measley Problem" appeared, another article is published in the *Philadelphia Inquirer* with a more sobering title: "Measles Deaths." The article warns that although the year hasn't reached its midpoint, the number of American children who have died from measles is more than that in all of 1989. The reason is that too many children are unimmunized. In response, the CDC changes its recommendation. Up to that point, children had received one dose of measles vaccine at fifteen months of age. Now, the CDC wants children to receive a second dose in middle school. The two-dose recommendation gives children a second chance to get their first vaccine. Also, whereas one dose of measles vaccine reduces the risk of disease by 95 percent, the additional dose reduces the risk by 99.5 percent—a level of protection that officials hope will put an end to this highly contagious disease.

Unfortunately, for the city of Philadelphia, it's too little too late.

Wednesday, January 16, 1991

Dr. Robert Ross, Philadelphia's Commissioner of Health, receives an anonymous phone call from a woman whose daughter belongs to the Faith Tabernacle Congregation in North Philadelphia. The woman warns that church members don't believe in medical care. "We nicknamed her Deep Throat," recalled Ross. "She was worried about her granddaughter because kids were getting sick in her school. No one had died yet. But for the first time we realized that we might not hear about a case of measles until a church parent calls the police or calls the coroner to pick up the body."

By November 29, 1990, measles has infected ninety-six Philadelphia children; by December 7, the number rises to 124; and by December 31, to 258. The 1990 outbreak is larger than anything the city has seen in more than a decade. Then, in December 1990, an eighteen-month-old unimmunized boy from North Philadelphia dies from measles pneumonia. It's the first time a Philadelphia resident has died from the disease in twenty years. One month later, in January 1991, another North Philadelphia child, also unimmunized, dies. In response, city health officials ask parents not to wait until their children are fifteen months old to vaccinate them. Instead, they recommend that all children receive the vaccine when they're six months old. "We want to get in and control it before things get much worse," says Dr. Robert Sharrar, assistant health commissioner for disease prevention.

Three weeks later, panicked by the number of children dying from measles, Philadelphia health officials do something that has never been done before—or since.

Thursday, February 7, 1991

After vomiting for four days, Caryn Still—a nine-year-old girl living on the 5200 block of North Howard Avenue—is taken by the Fire

Rescue Unit to Albert Einstein Hospital, where, at 8:21 P.M., she is pronounced dead. A third-grader, Caryn was one of hundreds of children who attend the Faith Tabernacle Congregation school. Because the church rejects all forms of modern medicine, not a single child in the school—which includes grades one through twelve—has been immunized. At the time of the outbreak, neither the church's pastor, Reverend Reinert, nor the associate pastor, Reverend Charles Kelly, grant interviews. This will soon change.

Faith Tabernacle's doctrine instructs members to "believe that the Bible is opposed to all means of healing apart from God's way." Church member Gordon Korn embraces this philosophy: "If I go to God and ask him to heal my body," he says, "I can't go to a doctor for medicine. You either trust God or you trust man." Recognizing that God's healing isn't foolproof, however, the church also teaches, "When we start out in naked faith, the Devil usually makes our symptoms worse and tries to persuade us to turn back from the Lord. But if we are steadfast, victory is sure." Caryn Still's death isn't the first time that Philadelphia's Faith Tabernacle Congregation has been in the news. In February 1990, Debra Still gave birth prematurely to twins in her Germantown home without the aid of a doctor or midwife. Both babies died. And in 1989, seventeen-year-old Leroy Carpenter Jr. died from a ruptured appendix after refusing surgery. Five years earlier, his fifteen-year-old sister, Lisa, died from untreated bacterial meningitis.

After Caryn Still dies from measles, Drs. Ross and Sharrar ask Reverend Reinert to immunize his students. Reinert refuses. "Sharrar and I visited Reinert," recalled Ross. "He was soft-spoken, the consummate gentlemen. But he drove us nuts. We told him we needed to vaccinate everyone in the school but he said the families wouldn't let us do it. We finally convinced Reinert to give us a list of the names and addresses of the families. We were used to people cooperating with us to stop the spread of disease. But he wouldn't cooperate."

Ross and Sharrar have no choice but to close the school—an action that will do nothing to slow the advancing epidemic.

SUNDAY, FEBRUARY 10, 1991

At 11:00 A.M., nine-year-old Monica Johnson, a classmate of Caryn Still's, is pronounced dead on arrival at the Medical College of Pennsylvania Hospital. Monica's illness began with a rash and progressed to labored breathing and unconsciousness. By the time the police arrived, her heart had stopped beating. Monica was one of eleven children in the home, all of whom had not been immunized. Her father, Wayne, a teacher at the Faith Tabernacle school, explains that his religion forbade him from calling a doctor when Monica had a rash, or when she had a high fever, or when she was gasping for air, or when she slipped into unconsciousness. It was only after she had stopped breathing that he called the police.

Wayne Johnson sees his ordeal as a test, "For the strengthening of our character," he says. "For the strengthening of our belief. That is why God has chosen her." He expresses no remorse for his part in his daughter's death. "I feel very confident in my belief in the way I've raised my children," he says. "[Monica] was something God has given us and now has taken away." Johnson's attitude shows public health officials just how hard it's going to be to get Philadelphia's measles outbreak under control. Some of Johnson's children are sick; others aren't. Those who aren't sick will clearly benefit from a measles vaccine. But Johnson is steadfast in his refusal to immunize them. "That's against my faith, immunization," he says. "It's interference with God's will."

Outside of Monica's home, a handful of young girls gather to remember their friend. Every weekend the girls would jump rope, play tag, and ride bikes. "I probably will never forget her smile because it always made me happy," says ten-year-old Kamilya Blackwell. "Even when she was sad, she had a smile."

TUESDAY, FEBRUARY 12, 1991

Health Commissioner Ross and public health nurse Hazel Gilstrop start calling Faith Tabernacle families. They ask parents whether their children have a rash, are holding down fluids, or are able to stand and walk. After telephoning dozens of families, they find that at least 129 students at Faith Tabernacle have come down with measles in the previous month. Only two families have no measles to report. Ross notes that parents are "articulate, intelligent, and calm," but "firm in their insistence that they will not allow their children to submit to medical care."

Ross and Gilstrop also find that none of the parents treat their children's fevers with Tylenol, which decreases the risk of dehydration. In fact, none of the parents own thermometers. Ross and Gilstrop are now worried about two groups: children who already have measles and might get sicker; and children who don't have the disease but remain at high risk because their parents refuse to immunize them.

WEDNESDAY, FEBRUARY 13, 1991

Ross obtains a court order to visit the families. "From what I heard on the telephone," he says, "it made sense to visit." Ross visits four homes and finds nine children with measles, none seriously ill. "The families were generally soft-spoken, pleasant, polite, regular people." But Ross is shaken by what he sees. "Most of these families had six, eight, ten, twelve kids because they didn't believe in birth control," he recalled. "There were also a lot of kids who were physically or developmentally disabled. They all had in-house deliveries. So if the kids were born breech [or with cords wrapped around their necks], they didn't do a Caesarian section. It was like the old days."

The parents are insistent, however, that Ross not be allowed to touch their children. He can only look at them through the doorway and in a glance try to figure out whether they are close to death. "These kids had the rash, they were lying in bed, but they were alert, conversant, and appeared to be well-hydrated," he says. "None appeared to need medical attention." Ross pleads with the parents to let him know if any of their children get sicker.

But he's whispering in the wind.

THURSDAY, FEBRUARY 14, 1991

On the morning of February 14, police are called to the two-story, colonial home of Linette Milnes, a fourteen-year-old girl with Down syndrome. Although Linette doesn't attend the Faith Tabernacle school, her sister does. The day before, Linette had had trouble breathing, so her parents sat up with her all night. By morning, according to Cheltenham detective sergeant Rich Hoffner, she is lifeless. An Emergency Medical Services team rushes her to Abington Hospital where, at 10:51 A.M., she is pronounced dead. Linette had seven brothers and sisters, all unimmunized.

Only three days earlier, Ross had called the Milnes's home. "When another kid turned up in the morgue I checked my list and realized she was on it," recalled Ross. "I had just called the mother and she told me her kids were fine. I thought, 'She lied to me! I just talked to this woman 48 hours ago!'" The case is referred to District Attorney Ronald Castille, who considers filing criminal charges, but demurs: "Unfortunately, when a parent is willing to risk the death of their children because of their religious beliefs, it's unlikely that the threat of prosecution will in any way act as a deterrent."

With the death of Linette Milnes, a line has been crossed. Ross now realizes that the information he is getting from parents is inaccurate, either because they can't tell whether their children are sick or, worse, because they are purposely misleading him so that he won't visit their homes. Either way, Ross changes his strategy. He obtains a court order permitting interns and residents at the two major children's hospitals in the city, St. Christopher's Hospital for Children and The Children's Hospital of Philadelphia, to go door-to-door. This time, however, doctors aren't going to stand in the doorway and peek in; now, they can physically examine the children. "I said I needed a bunch of doctors to see these kids," recalled Ross. "It was one of the more inspiring moments in my thirty years in healthcare to see how the residents, fellows, and faculty members rallied. These are busy people, on call every third night, and yet they were only too happy to do it."

Ross talks to Mayor Wilson Goode, hoping to take the next step. "I asked the mayor if we could get the city attorney to get us a court order in case any of these children looked bad enough to be hospitalized." Goode agrees. "We recognize that this is a First Amendment issue, which must be balanced with public health concerns," says Goode. "We are prepared, however, to ask the court to intervene in the lives of at-risk children."

"Everything has a context," recalled Ross. "Goode had a calm, professional demeanor, but the idea that these kids were dying on the front page of the newspaper and that our system was virtually powerless to stop it really bothered him. I could tell he was haunted by the MOVE bombing." (In the spring of 1985, a back-to-nature group called MOVE took over a house in West Philadelphia. The group had long been a nuisance to the city, with members assaulting neighbors, ignoring sanitation codes, and shouting through megaphones late into the night. During one police raid, an officer was shot and killed. On May 13, 1985, police dropped an improvised bomb on top of the house. The explosion killed eleven people, including five children, and burned down an entire city block. Wilson Goode's administration never fully recovered.)

Following the court order, visiting doctors are given the telephone number of a judge should legal action be needed for any child requiring hospitalization. Stethoscopes, ophthalmoscopes, otoscopes, and black bags in hand, the doctors visit the homes of more than four hundred children who are members of the Faith Tabernacle Congregation, hoping to prevent what has happened to Caryn Still, Monica Johnson, and Linette Milnes. Heading the St. Christopher's team is Dr. Mark Joffe, director of emergency services. Joffe notes that he is probably the first doctor these parents have ever seen. "It was like entering a time warp," he says. Joffe finds that parents are "extremely courteous, caring and honest," but he can't ignore the elephant in the room. "With the exception of the fact that they stay at home and watch their children die of measles," he says, "they seem like wonderful people." Dr. Maura Cooper heads The Children's Hospital of Philadelphia team. "It was definitely different than anything the [pediatric] residents had experienced," says Cooper. "It's not that the children are not well cared for. It's just that these are huge families with no access to medical care. You wonder about the stress of taking care of thirteen kids who were all sick in a three-week time span."

Friday, February 15, 1991

Early in the morning, Nancy Evans, a five-year-old girl who lives in North Central Philadelphia, is pronounced dead from measles. Nancy isn't a student of the Faith Tabernacle school; she's a member of the First-Century Gospel Church, another Philadelphia fundamentalist church that rejects modern medicine. A few hours later, thirteen-year-old Tina Louise Johnson dies from measles. Tina, the sister of Monica Johnson, dies on the day of Monica's funeral. Not surprisingly, neither of these children has been immunized and neither had been taken to a doctor when their illnesses worsened.

Five children have died in ten days. Philadelphia is in the midst of the worst measles epidemic in US history. Typically, about one of every one thousand children with measles dies from the disease. Sometimes, the death rate can reach as high as one in three hundred. But in Philadelphia in February of 1991, 4 of the 150 children with measles whose parents attend a single church are dead. That's a death rate of one in thirty-five, worse than that found in any developing world country.

The CDC sends a team of scientists to Philadelphia. Dr. William Atkinson, who heads the investigation, wants to find out why the death rate is so high. He considers the possibility that the circulating strain of measles is particularly virulent. But Atkinson finds that the measles deaths have nothing to do with the virus and everything to do with the parents. Children aren't dying because of a unique strain; they're dying because they're not getting intravenous fluids for their dehydration or oxygen for their pneumonia. Worse, about sixty healthy, unimmunized children are still living in the homes of other children with measles. And their parents are refusing to get medical care—a recipe for more deaths.

Public opinion has turned against the Faith Tabernacle Congregation and its members. But Reverend Reinert refuses to compromise his most fundamental belief. Angry that the press has accused his congregation of being a cult, Reinert strikes back. "The Devil has tried to put fear in people's hearts," he says. "Job was robbed of everything he had. He was smitten with sores. As he went through that trial he learned through it. There is no fear when you can see God on your side." Reinert interprets the deaths of children in his congregation as a test of faith—a test he and his fellow church members have every intention of passing. "It's drawing us all together as one body," he says.

Saturday, February 16, 1991

When members of the Faith Tabernacle Congregation allowed doctors to call or visit their homes, they could argue that they still hadn't received medical care. Now, however, public health officials are insisting that sick children be hospitalized, independent of their parents' beliefs.

On February 16, a physician working for the Philadelphia health department examines four-year-old Daniel Kirn in Northeast Philadelphia. Kirn, who has measles virus pneumonia, is getting worse. The doctor advises the Kirns to take their son to a hospital. If they don't, he insists, Daniel is in danger of dying "in the next twenty-four hours." The parents "politely but firmly" refuse. So, Health Commissioner Ross calls City Solicitor Charisse Lille, who calls Family Court Judge Edward Summers, who issues an emergency order to hospitalize the boy.

Sunday, February 17, 1991

Against his parents' wishes, Daniel Kirn is taken to St. Christopher's Hospital. "It was done rather peacefully," says Ross. Later in the day, the parents of a second child, two-year-old Bianca Carpena, are also advised to take their daughter to an emergency room. Because the Carpenas "did not want someone to take their child away," they agree. But when the emergency department physician tells them that Bianca needs to be hospitalized, they refuse. A second court order is obtained, and Bianca is admitted.

Ross REMEMBERED ONE telling moment. "So I go to this last house on my list and the grandmother answers the door. The parents were both at work. There were nine kids on my list. I walk in and most of these kids are bouncing around, playing, and reading. But I only see eight kids. I ask where is the ninth child. She tells me she's upstairs watching TV and she's fine. I ask her if she minds if I look at her real quick. She says she does mind but she lets me follow her upstairs. The kid is propped up on pillows in front of the television: ashen, gray, pale, clammy, glassy eyed, not very responsive, and hyperventilating. She looks like hell. So I run downstairs to call the judge and the grandmother is trying to physically restrain me from dialing the phone. She's yelling at me, 'Don't you believe in the power of the Lord! Don't you believe that Jesus heals all! Your medicine can't help her!' She's yelling this in my ear while I'm talking to the judge. I'm six feet two inches and this woman's five feet tall and maybe ninety pounds. The judge gives the order, the paramedics show up, they put her on the bus [ambulance], wheel her off, and she goes to St. Christopher's Hospital where she's diagnosed with pneumonia. The next morning I wanted to see how she was doing so I went to St. Chris's intensive care unit. She looks 100 percent better. She's on facemask oxygen. But she's got color; she's alert. When I saw the parents I was expecting them to say, 'Thank you, she looks so much better today.' But all I got was a room full of cold, icy stares."

THE MEASLES EPIDEMIC IN Philadelphia is now at its peak. At Children's Hospital of Philadelphia, eighty-two children have been treated in the emergency department and twenty-eight have been hospitalized. At St. Christopher's Hospital, which is closer to the homes of church members, 250 children have been treated in the emergency department and three are being hospitalized every week. Ross and his team have visited eighty families and examined almost five hundred children. Most of the children have either fully recovered or are on their way to recovering. But some have yet to become ill. "There will be more measles deaths in the city of Philadelphia," says Ross.

DURING THE TRAGEDY, Robert Ross is forced to confront his faith. "This thing caught me at a time when I was really at odds with organized religion," he recalled. "I grew up Catholic and religion had always been an important part of my life. But starting around med school and for about a decade I stopped going to church and became estranged from the faith I'd grown up in. When the Faith Tabernacle thing hit, I found myself simultaneously infuriated with the leadership of the church and oddly in awe at the strength of their beliefs. I wished I had a fraction of the belief in the higher power that these people had." Ironically, in the midst of the outbreak, Ross found himself in church: "I remember in the middle of it, after the second or third death, I went to a Catholic church near City Hall. I sat in the front pew. It was the first time I'd been in church in a long time. I found myself praying for guidance because I just felt so lost. And I remember a sense of solace from that spiritual moment. And I remember thinking how odd it was that what had driven these kids to their death was this undying, unyielding faith, which was the very issue we were fighting against. Yet at that moment I needed a dose of spirituality to give me an inspiration to help me figure out what to do."

TUESDAY, FEBRUARY 19, 1991

A court order is obtained to hospitalize two girls, ages one and nine, who are suffering from measles pneumonia. Four children have been hospitalized under court order.

Philadelphia is now a feared destination. Two nearby schools cancel trips to the city.

THURSDAY, FEBRUARY 21, 1991

Under siege by the press and the public, Reverend Reinert issues a statement. He admits that the measles deaths in his congregation have been "a little wearing." But he is confident that the faith of church members has grown even stronger. "There's been a real cleaning up in our midst," he says. "All four of those funeral bills have been paid for. That's how our people stand together."

THE MEASLES OUTBREAK in Philadelphia has taken a financial toll. "Everyone in this department put in extra hours, even on the weekend and holiday weeks," says Robert Levenson, director of the Health Department's division of disease control. The city has authorized overtime hours, filled previously unfilled positions, solicited help from the Visiting Nurses Association of Philadelphia, printed fifty thousand educational pamphlets, and vaccinated hundreds of preschool children every week in an attempt to stem the tide. In support, the commonwealth of Pennsylvania has sent $100,000 in federal funds to keep the city's health clinics open on Saturdays. But health officials know that if children in the Faith Tabernacle and First-Century Gospel churches remain unimmunized, they're still at risk. And the city is growing increasingly tired of trying to prevent deaths by daily home visits. Health officials are ready to take the final step—to force children to be vaccinated against their parents' will.

REVEREND REINERT AND MEMBERS of his congregation would probably have been surprised to learn that—as a result of two critical rulings by the United States Supreme Court—states have the legal right to compel people to be vaccinated during outbreaks.

In the early 1900s, a smallpox epidemic swept through Cambridge, Massachusetts. The Cambridge Board of Public Health asked citizens to receive a smallpox vaccine; if not, they had to pay a five-dollar fine. Henning Jacobson, a Lutheran minister, believing that God would protect him, refused both. His case eventually went to the United States Supreme Court, where he lost. "The liberty secured by the Constitution of the United States," wrote Associate

Justice John Marshall Harlan, "does not import an absolute right to be wholly freed from restraint. There are manifold restraints to which every person is necessarily subject for the common good. Society based on the rule that each one is a law unto himself would soon be confronted with anarchy and disorder."

Seventeen years later, the United States Supreme Court revisited its ruling in *Jacobson v. Massachusetts*. In the early 1920s, after refusing a smallpox vaccine, Rosalyn Zucht was expelled from Brackenridge High School in San Antonio, Texas. Like Henning Jacobson's case, Zucht's case also worked its way up to the Supreme Court. The difference between the Zucht and Jacobson cases was that, unlike Cambridge, San Antonio wasn't in the midst of a smallpox epidemic. So Rosalyn's risk of catching smallpox was small. Nevertheless, the Supreme Court, in a one-paragraph opinion, upheld the previous ruling.

And that was that. The United States Supreme Court has ruled on the issue of using religion as a justification for avoiding vaccination twice; both times, the Court ruled in support of a state's right to compel vaccination. States can, however, enact laws that ignore these Supreme Court rulings. During the 1960s and 1970s, several parents argued before state supreme courts that their First Amendment right to practice religion freely should include the right to avoid vaccination. Each time they lost, the courts ruled that because states were asking *everyone* to be vaccinated, parents weren't being persecuted on the basis of their religion; all religions were being treated equally.

In the mid-1960s, however, a door opened. On June 20, 1966, New York State legislators, by a vote of 150 to 2, passed a bill requiring polio vaccine for school entry. The two dissenters were concerned about a clause that excluded parents whose religion forbade vaccination—a clause that had been added because of the successful lobbying efforts of Christian Scientists. Now there was a state law that allowed parents to opt out of vaccines on the basis of their religion.

The predictable happened. A few years later, an outbreak of polio in a Christian Science school paralyzed eleven children. Because polio paralyzes fewer than 1 percent of those infected—and because 128 children attended the school—it was likely that every child in the school had been infected with the virus. In response to this outbreak, a local health official wrote, "I am deeply bothered that disease-prevention measures of documented benefit can be withheld by their parents in the name of religious freedoms, jeopardizing the health of the community as well. The courts of this land have long since set precedent in the protection of children from the irresponsible acts of their parents."

The New York State law changed everything. Now, parents could argue that they were being discriminated against because they *weren't* Christian Scientists. As a consequence, forty-one states now allow religious exemptions to vaccination. Pennsylvania is one of them. So, when Health Commissioner Robert Ross and Mayor Wilson Goode tried to force members of the Faith Tabernacle and First-Century Gospel churches to receive a measles vaccine, they were running headlong into a law that had been on the books for more than a decade.

WEDNESDAY, FEBRUARY 27, 1991

Mayor Wilson Goode directs the City Solicitor's office to obtain a court order to forcibly vaccinate children. "We have children dying," says Goode, "and every conceivable step must be taken to prevent any further loss of life."

Goode has crossed the line from mandatory vaccination to compulsory vaccination. Mandatory vaccination requires people to receive a vaccine or pay some sort of societal price, such as a fine (as was the case for Henning Jacobson), or being excluded from school (as was the case for Rosalyn Zucht). Compulsory vaccination, on the other hand, requires people to be vaccinated whether they want to be or not. In the 250-year history of the United States, no child had been vaccinated against his or her parents' will. "As far as I can tell," says William Atkinson, head of the measles surveillance team for the CDC, "this is precedent setting." Reverend Reinert, on the other hand, is appalled. "It's persecution," he says. "We remain committed to God, the supreme justice of the universe."

Friday, March 1, 1991

Reverend Reinert asks lawyers from the American Civil Liberties Union (ACLU) to represent his church in its fight against compulsory vaccination. In picking the ACLU, Reinert chooses an organization that has a long history of representing controversial and unpopular causes, right up to the present day. For example:

In 2009, the ACLU of Florida filed a lawsuit on behalf of the families of children from the Dove World Outreach Center, defending their constitutional right to wear T-shirts to school stating, "Islam Is Of The Devil." Saeed Khan, president of the Muslim Association of North Central Florida, was upset by the shirts, and pleased when the school prohibited students from wearing them. ACLU lawyers, however, chose to represent the students, telling Khan that while it didn't agree with what the shirts said, it supported the students' right to say it. "As far as we are concerned, they are condoning [the shirts] with this lawsuit," said Khan. "Some of the parents who spoke to the school board told them that our children were waking up in the middle of the night, unable to sleep, and asking 'Why don't they like us?'" The ACLU won the right of students to wear the hateful shirts to school.

In 2007, the ACLU defended the right of Shirley Phelps-Roper to protest at the site of funerals. Phelps-Roper was a member of a Topeka, Kansas, church that believed that God was punishing America for allowing the sin of homosexuality. (The Westboro Baptist

Church's website is godhatesfags.com.) The punishment that God had chosen, according to Phelps-Roper, was the killing of American soldiers. "While we disagree with the message that tolerance of gay people has corrupted America," said Anthony Rothert, legal director of the ACLU of Eastern Missouri, "it is not the job of government to silence speech that we don't want to hear." The ACLU won the case, and Phelps-Roper continued to disrupt funerals, including those of soldiers who had recently died in Iraq.

Most famously, in 1977, the ACLU defended the right of the National Socialist Party of America, a neo-Nazi group based in Chicago, to march down the streets of Skokie, Illinois: a town that since World War II had become the center of Chicago's Jewish community, including many Holocaust survivors. The ACLU won the case when the Illinois Appellate Court declared that the march, the anti-Semitic speeches, and the public display of Nazi swastikas were within the bounds of free speech. (The ACLU's penchant for taking on outrageous cases has been easy to satirize. In 2003, the humorous online news source *The Onion* wrote an article titled "ACLU Defends Nazi's Right to Burn Down ACLU Headquarters.")

When Reverend Reinert asked the ACLU of Pennsylvania to defend his church's right to refuse vaccines—a right that had been afforded by state law—everyone assumed that ACLU lawyers would rush to his defense. But the ACLU declined. "There is certainly a free exercise of religion claim by the parents," said Deborah Levy, executive director of the Philadelphia chapter of the ACLU, "but there is also a competing claim that parents don't have the right to martyr their children. I don't think we've walked away from our principles here." Jim Crawford, chairman of the board of the Philadelphia ACLU, agreed. "We just don't want to find ourselves taking the position that the city has to allow children to get good and sick before it has the right to intervene."

MONDAY, MARCH 4, 1991

Family Court Judge Edward R. Summers orders city officials to disregard the state rule allowing a religious exemption to vaccination. Six children whose parents are members of the Faith Tabernacle Congregation will now temporarily become wards of the court and will be given the measles vaccine. Summers orders the children to be vaccinated within the week.

Jerome Balter, a lawyer for the parents, appeals the decision. Balter says that "their healing is dependent on their faith; they believe that's the way to do right by their children." Health Commissioner Ross, on the other hand, is tired of chasing sick children around the city, preferring to protect them from getting sick rather than waiting until they're sick to treat them. And he no longer trusts the parents of Faith Tabernacle. "No one has ever called us to say their kids were sick," he says. "In every case we had to go out to families and call and visit. And, quite frankly, this is no way to run an operation. I just don't want them to get sick. This is not what I learned about in med school."

FRIDAY, MARCH 8, 1991

State Superior Court Judge Vincent A. Cirillo hears the appeal of the decision by Family Court Judge Edward Summers to compel vaccination. Again, Jerome Balter is representing the parents; Shawn Lacy is the public defender representing the children. Cirillo, noticing a look on Lacy's face, stops the proceedings. "Are you ill?" he asks. Lacy has just been handed a note stating that twenty-month-old James Jones, whose parents belong to Faith Tabernacle, died at 9:30 that morning. Jones's mother had told physicians who called her home that her son was fine; but the father later admitted that the boy had had a fever and a rash. Unknown to the parents, James also had measles encephalitis. By the time he was brought to the hospital, he was brain dead.

James Jones is the fifth Faith Tabernacle child to die from measles. Word of his death freezes the hearing. Balter temporarily halts his argument. When he continues, he says that parents are now willing to have their children examined and hospitalized as long as they don't have to be vaccinated. Balter implies that treatment is at least as good as prevention, an argument contradicted by events of the previous two weeks.

Within an hour, Cirillo rejects the appeal and orders six children to be vaccinated. The judge praises the parents for "adhering to the Good Book" and calls them "good people," but in the end he rules that religious freedoms aren't absolute.

Balter asks the State Supreme Court to invalidate Cirillo's ruling, but the Court refuses to intervene.

Health Commissioner Ross administers measles vaccine to six children at an undisclosed location. Parents, grandparents, and church elders are present. Everyone is described as "fully cooperative."

FRIDAY, MARCH 15, 1991

Family Court Judge Edward Summers orders a second round of vaccines for children of the Faith Tabernacle school. Lawyers for the parents don't bother to fight it. "Why go through the same deal again?" says Balter. "A precedent has been set. I don't think any court is going to come up with a different answer."

FRIDAY, JUNE 7, 1991

The measles epidemic of Philadelphia subsides. "Typically measles is a disease of late winter and early spring," says Robert Levenson, director of the city's division of disease control. "When the spring and warm weather comes, the cases disappear." Reverend Reinert has a different interpretation. Ignoring the fact that almost everyone in his congregation had been previously infected, recently infected, hospitalized, or killed by the measles virus—and that the death rate from measles in his congregation was astronomical—he claims that, in the end, faith in the Lord allowed the remaining children in his flock to survive. "We believe God has provided his faithfulness," he declares.

THURSDAY, DECEMBER 3, 1992

Almost two years after the outbreak in Philadelphia subsides, CDC investigators submit their final report.

The Faith Tabernacle Congregation and the First-Century Gospel Church were at the center of an outbreak in Philadelphia that affected more than 1,400 people. Among church members, 486 people were infected and six were killed by measles. Among non-church members, 938 people were infected and three were killed. All nine fatalities were children. Because they hadn't been vaccinated, the attack rate among church members was a thousand times higher than that in the surrounding community.

IN 2013, THE CDC identified thirty thousand children whose parents had chosen not to vaccinate them for religious reasons. Given the degree of underreporting and the insular nature of some of these religious groups, the actual number of children at risk is likely far greater.

8

UNGODLY ACTS

"The healing ministry of Jesus is one of the best evidences
of the love of God that I know."

—Père Jean Leclerq,
Benedictine scholar

In 1984, Gary and Margaret Hall refused antibiotics for their twenty-six-day-old son, Joel, who suffered from pneumonia. Members of the Faith Assembly Church in Indiana, they chose prayer instead. Joel died as a result. Margaret was unrepentant. Clutching her Bible, she said, "When our little son, Joel, was sick, I didn't take him to a medical doctor. I took him to Jesus, who is our doctor, to heal him. The Bible didn't change because of what happened. I still believe that Jesus is our doctor and that he desires us to trust in him no matter what happens."

Faith healing parents often argue that they were only doing what Jesus would have done. But what would He have done?—this man who dedicated his life to relieving the illness, poverty, and death around him; who wept at the suffering of children; who stood up for those who couldn't stand up for themselves. One can only imagine Jesus would have used whatever was available to prevent that suffering, much as Christians have been doing in His name for centuries.

AT THE TIME OF JESUS'S BIRTH, several religions were dominant in Persia, Egypt, and Greece. Although they centered on different gods who did different things, all shared the same belief about what caused disease. People were sick because the gods had punished them for their sins. If they wanted to be cured, they had to repent. Healers were shamans, witches, and priests; treatments were prayers, sacrifices, and exorcisms.

Unlike other dominant religions, Judaism didn't embrace multiple gods (polytheism); it embraced one God (monotheism). But it still believed that people got sick because they'd done something wrong. The Old Testament is full of stories of God punishing those who had offended Him. When Miriam slandered Moses, she was stricken with leprosy (Numbers 12:10). When the Egyptians were hard hearted, they suffered ten plagues including lice, pestilence, boils, and death of their first-born children (Exodus 8:12–13; 9:2–6; 9:8–10; 12:29). When David took a forbidden census of his people, God gave him a choice of famine, conquest, or plague. David chose plague, and God killed seventy thousand Israelites (1 Chronicles 21:1–14).

JESUS WAS BORN A JEW. His Hebrew name was Yeshua ben Yosef (Joshua, the son of Joseph). But Jesus's views of illness and healing were *not* those of his faith. Several religious scholars have argued that Jesus's beliefs were influenced by one story in the Old Testament that stands apart from the rest—a story that Jesus probably heard as a child.

There was a man in the land of Uz, whose name was Job, the story begins. Job was a prosperous man. He enjoyed the love of his wife, three daughters, and seven sons. And he owned thousands of sheep, oxen, and cattle. Most importantly, he *was whole-hearted and upright, and one that feared God and shunned evil.*

But Job was about to be the unknowing victim of a bet between God and the Devil. *Now it fell upon a day, that the sons of God came to present themselves before the Lord and Satan came also along with them.* God asked Satan what he'd been doing; Satan said he'd been *going to and fro in the earth.* Curious, God asked Satan whether he'd encountered Job in his wanderings, a man whom God considered pious, humble, and without sin. *'Hast thou considered My servant Job,' asked God, 'that there is none like him in the earth?'* The Devil wasn't impressed, reasoning that it was much easier to respect God if you were rich and had a large family than if you were poor and alone. *'Doth Job fear God for naught?'* asked the Devil. *'Hast Thou not made a hedge about him, and about his house, and about all that he hath, on every side? Thou hast blessed the work of his hands, and his possessions are increased in the land.'*

The Devil bet that if Job lost his great wealth, he would surely renounce God. *'Put forth Thy hand now,'* said the Devil, *'and touch all that he hath; surely he will blaspheme Thee to Thy face.'* The bet in place, *Satan went forth from the presence of the Lord.*

First the Devil took away Job's possessions. A raid by the Sabeans killed Job's oxen, donkeys, and servants. Then a *fire from heaven* burned all his sheep. Then a raid by the Chaldeans killed all his camels. Then *a great wind from across the wilderness* killed Job's children. Despite these misfortunes, Job didn't renounce God. *'Naked came I out of my mother's womb,'* said Job, *'and naked shall I return thither; the Lord gave, and the Lord hath taken away; blessed be the name of the Lord.'*

Despite Job's unwavering faith, the Devil wasn't ready to admit defeat, arguing that Job hadn't renounced God because he hadn't suffered physically. *'Put forth Thy hand now,'* said the Devil, *'and touch his bone and his flesh; surely he will blaspheme Thee to Thy face.'* *The Lord said to Satan, 'Behold, he is in thy hand; only spare his life.'* So *Satan went forth from the presence of the Lord, and smote Job with sore boils from the sole of his foot even unto his crown. And* [Job] *took him a potsherd* [a fragment of broken pottery] *to scrape himself therewith;*

and he sat among the ashes. Job's wife wasn't particularly supportive, telling Job to *'blaspheme God and die.'* But Job didn't relent, saying, *'What? Shall we receive good at the hand of God, and shall we not receive evil?'*

Later, three friends visited Job—all assuming that he had done something horribly wrong to warrant such suffering. One said, *'They that plow iniquity, and sow mischief, reap the same. By the breath of God they perish. And by the blast of His anger are they consumed.'*

Job was unfazed, continuing to praise God. In the end, the Devil relented and *the Lord gave Job twice as much as he had before. And after this Job lived a hundred and forty years and saw his sons and his sons' sons, even four generations. So Job died, being old and full of days.*

The Book of Job contradicts much of what the Old Testament teaches about why people get sick. Job suffers boils even though he hadn't sinned against God; quite the opposite, he'd been God's loyal servant.

WHILE RELIGIOUS HEALING isn't part of the Jewish tradition, it was at the very heart of Jesus's ministry. The New Testament includes forty-one separate instances of healing. Of the 3,779 verses in the four gospels, 727 relate specifically to healing. In other words, one-fifth of all the gospel writings tell of Jesus's miraculous power to heal. Jesus cured leprosy, paralysis, dropsy, fever, and epilepsy. He caused the deaf to hear and the mute to speak. He cured withered hands and severed ears. He presided over mass healings, in which all who touched him were made whole. And he did it by talking, exorcism, "laying on of the hands," and saliva, either alone or mixed with mud. Sometimes Jesus healed by allowing sufferers to simply touch the hem of his garment. (Of interest, Jesus never healed the sick by anointing them with oil; only his disciples did that.) Healing was so important to Jesus that he did it during the Sabbath, when he wasn't supposed to work.

Several of Jesus's encounters were particularly instructive. When Jesus was confronted with the suffering of the Galileans, he said, *'Do you suppose these Galileans who suffered like that were greater sinners than any other Galileans? They were not, I tell you. Or those eighteen on whom the tower at Siloam fell and killed them? Do you suppose that they were guiltier than all the other people living in Jerusalem? They were not, I tell you'* (Luke 13:2–5). And when he was questioned about a man born blind, he said, *'Neither he nor his parents sinned'* and added, *'he was born blind so that the works of God might be displayed in him'* (John 9:3). Jesus's strongly held belief that disease was arbitrary—occurring in equal measure in the virtuous and sinful—put him in direct conflict with the religion of his people.

According to Jesus, illness was the result of bad luck, not bad acts. Nowhere in the gospels does Jesus ask people what they had done wrong to become ill. Jesus's ministry was evidence that God cared about those who suffered. *'if it is through the spirit of God that I cast devils out,'* he said, *'then know that the kingdom of God has overtaken you'* (Matthew 12:27–28). Jesus wasn't hostile to people who were sick. He was hostile to the forces that had made them sick.

Jesus embraced a modern concept of disease. When people are admitted to the hospital with a serious illness, doctors don't assume they've done something wrong, something to evoke God's anger. Rather, they interpret illness as a problem within the patient, not divine retribution from without. Jesus wasn't the first to advance this notion. The Greek healer Hippocrates—who lived four hundred years before Jesus—argued that disease was caused by an imbalance of internal "humors" that he called yellow bile, black bile, phlegm, and blood. Because Hippocrates was the first to propose that internal physical processes, not God, cause disease, he's called the "Father of Modern Medicine." But Jesus took Hippocrates's idea one step further, adding love and compassion to the healing process. "It has become traditional to identify modern doctors in spirit with a long line of historic greats reaching back to the impressive Hippocrates," writes Dr. Jack Provonsha, professor of philosophy of religion at Loma Linda University. "This notable Greek, a veritable pinnacle in ancient medicine, often called 'The Father of Medicine,' largely set the pattern for current professional attitudes and relationships. But sometimes it is forgotten that medicine owes its greatest debt not to Hippocrates, but to Jesus. It was the humble Galilean who more than any other figure in history bequeathed to the healing arts its essential meaning and spirit. Jesus brings to methods and codes the corrective love without which true healing is rarely actually possible. The spiritual 'Father of Medicine' was not Hippocrates of the island of Cos, but Jesus of the town of Nazareth!"

Most importantly, Jesus embraced doctors. Nowhere in the New Testament is Jesus hostile to the medicine of his time. *'It is not the healthy who need a doctor,' said Jesus, 'but the sick'* (Matthew 9:12; Mark 2:17; Luke 5:31). "There is the idea among Christians that Jesus came to provide a do-it-yourself manual for human beings," writes biblical scholar Morton Kelsey, "that his primary purpose was to teach ingenuity, self-reliance, and the one right method of spiritual healing so as to avoid sickness. This does not tally with the record. [Jesus] made *no* explicit suggestion that people should learn to get along without physicians. [Rather] Jesus dignified intelligence as a way for humankind to deal with their problems."

What all of this means is that when faith-healing parents perceive their children's illnesses to be a test of their faith, they have ignored the essence of Jesus's ministry. "The coming of Jesus," writes Kelsey, "wipes out once and for all the notion that God puts sickness upon people because of Divine Will." What kind of God, asks Kelsey, would give a child meningitis, diabetes, or cancer as a test of faith?

INFLUENCED BY THE TEACHINGS of Jesus, early Christians set a standard for how medicine should be practiced.

In the second century AD, Polycarp, Bishop of Smyrna, identified care of the sick as a principal responsibility of church elders. Indeed, according to Amanda Porterfield in *Healing in Early Christianity*, "early Christians nursed the sick to emulate the healing ministry of Jesus, to express their faith in the ongoing healing power of Christ, and to distinguish Christian heroism in the face of sickness and death from pagan fear."

By the end of the third century, no single entity had advanced healing more than monasteries, which treated the sick, disabled, and elderly. And they didn't rely on prayer alone to do it; they relied on doctors and nurses. Christian monasteries—which put inpatient and outpatient care into a single building—gave birth to the modern-day hospital. By the Middle Ages, Christians had created more hospitals than any other religious or secular entity.

Christian monasteries inspired Christian missionaries, who were often the first to bring modern medicine to many parts of the world. And as medicine had more to offer, missionaries had greater influence. Indeed, medical missionaries often imagined that Jesus might have been one of them—perhaps no one more so than the most famous missionary of them all: Albert Schweitzer, who, in the name of Jesus, brought vaccines, antibiotics, anesthetics, and surgery to a small part of Africa in the early 1900s.

Schweitzer wasn't alone. Christian missionaries have brought the latest medical advances to virtually every part of the globe. The United Church Mission Hospitals have been training medical students and serving remote areas in Canada for more than 115 years. And missionaries were the backbone of the medical infrastructure in China prior to the revolution, establishing two hundred nursing schools. Edward Bliss, an American missionary who worked in China for most of his life, saw his work as "the embodiment of the Divine Idea." Bliss built a hospital and dispensary in Shaowu and fought *rinderpest*, a virus that decimated cattle. In 1922, Bliss wrote,

"God had an only Son, and He was a missionary and a physician. A poor, poor imitation of Him I am, or hope to be. In this service I hope to live; in it I wish to die."

IN THE UNITED STATES, the influence of Jesus's teachings is also apparent. The entrance to Pennsylvania Hospital in Philadelphia—the first hospital built in the United States—bears the image of the Good Samaritan along with the phrase *take care of him and I will repay thee* (Luke 10:35). Of the six thousand hospitals in the United States, religious groups support more than one in ten. And although it has wrestled with issues of abortion and reproductive rights, no religious or secular entity has embraced and advanced the practice of modern medicine more than the Catholic health-care system.

Still, although Jesus was in many ways a spiritual inspiration for today's healers, some people choose to reject modern therapies and allow children to die in His name. The irony doesn't end there. Allowing children to suffer in the name of Jesus is inconceivable for another reason; it relates to how children were treated at the time of Jesus's birth—and to how Jesus responded to what he saw.

IN THE EARLY 1900s, excavations at Gezer—a biblical town in ancient Israel—unearthed a disturbing artifact: jars containing the bones of newborn babies. These jars were found within the foundations of buildings—each containing food for the next life. "None were over a week old," said Stewart MacAlistar, who was in charge of the excavations. "The sacrifices were not offered under stress or any special calamity, or at the rites attached to any special season of the year. The only cause most likely to be in effect was primogeniture." First-born children had been killed, put in jars, and buried as good-luck charms for building occupants. Archaeologists call them "foundation sacrifices."

A few years later, excavations at Ta'Anneck, not far from Gezer, unearthed more children, also buried in jars; this time, children as old as five years had been killed. Ancient foundation sacrifices, which date back to the walls of Jericho in 7,000 BC (Joshua 6:26; 1 Kings 16:34), have also been found in India, New Zealand, China, Japan, Mexico, Germany, and Denmark.

AT THE TIME OF JESUS'S BIRTH, infanticide was legal. Children weren't considered to be people; they were property, no different than slaves. So parents could do whatever they wanted to them. Children were stoned, beaten, flung into dung heaps, starved to death, traded for beds, sexually abused, sold into slavery, and "exposed on every hill and roadside as prey for birds and food for wild beasts." Some boys were killed so that their livers, brains, testicles, and bone marrow could be used in love potions. When children had nightmares, they were beaten to drive the devils out. For entertainment, girls were raped and children were suspended on poles so that hyenas could tear them apart. When the Emperor Diocletian fell ill in AD 303, anyone who didn't sacrifice a child was immediately executed. Infanticide—an everyday occurrence—was, according to one historian, "the most widely used method of population control during much of human history."

Although illegitimate, deformed, and disabled children were particularly vulnerable, no group suffered more than young girls. And it didn't matter whether parents were rich or poor, times were good or bad, or children were healthy or sick; girls were often the first to be killed. Pagan Arabs buried their infant daughters alive. For convenience, mothers gave birth in a pit; sons were saved; daughters were buried.

Female infanticides were so common that they caused an imbalance in the ratio of boys to girls. In 220 BC, among seventy-nine families in Melitus (a city in modern-day Turkey), there were 118 sons but only 28 daughters. Many families had two sons, some had three, but none had more than one daughter. Of six hundred families found on second-century inscriptions at Delphi, only 1 percent raised two daughters.

INFANTICIDES WEREN'T A SECRET. The Old Testament is filled with stories of ritual child murder, the best known being that of Abraham's willingness to sacrifice Isaac.

Although Abraham was upset when God asked him to take his only son up to Mount Moriah and stab him to death, he wasn't surprised by the request and proceeded with the execution in a business-like manner. But God stayed his hand (Genesis 22:11–12). For Abraham, the concept of child sacrifice was familiar territory; he, too, had been saved by God's intervention. After Abraham's mother had abandoned him in a cave, God had sent the angel Gabriel to nurture him.

Moses was also spared. The Old Testament tells of an unnamed Egyptian Pharaoh who ordered the slaying of all Hebrew male children by drowning them in the river Nile. Instead of letting Moses be drowned, his mother, Jochebed, set him adrift in the river in a small craft made of bulrushes coated in pitch. Eventually, Moses was spotted by Pharaoh's daughter, who raised him as her son (Exodus 1:15–22; 2:1–10).

In fact, the concept of Hell was inspired by a real place—a region where children were routinely burned to death. The New Testament reference to Hell is Gehenna, a colloquialization of Ge-Hinnom. Called the "valley of slaughter" by Jeremiah, Hinnom isn't far from Jerusalem (Jeremiah 7:32). Several kings sacrificed children to gods whose shrines had been built there (2 Chronicles 28:3, 33:6). Ironically, the valley of Hinnom (called Guy Ben Hinnom today) was later turned into a garbage dump that burned continuously, providing the image of the fires of Hell.

So common was child sacrifice at the time of Jesus that everyone—including academics, historians, and physicians—accepted it. In Athens, a cultured city alive with artists, poets, architects, and philosophers, starving and dying children were objects of humor. Plato and Aristotle both believed that killing deformed children was necessary for society to function. And Seneca, a Roman statesman, dramatist, and advisor to the emperor Nero, argued that parents who mutilated their children had done them a favor. "Look on the blind wandering about the streets leaning on their sticks, and those with crushed feet," he wrote, "and still again look on those with broken limbs. This one is without arms, that one has had his shoulder pulled down out of shape in order that his grotesqueness may excite laughter. Each has a different profession; a different mutilation has given each a different occupation. What wrong has been done to the republic? On the contrary, have not these children been done a service?" William Lecky, an Irish historian, has called infanticide and child abuse "the crying vice of the Roman empire."

Even the Hippocratic Oath, written as a guide for physicians in the fifth century BC, doesn't protect children. "Whenever I go into a house," wrote Hippocrates, "I will go to help the sick and never with the intention of doing harm or injury. I will not abuse my position [of authority] to indulge in sexual contacts with the bodies of men or women, whether they be freemen or slaves." Hippocrates never mentioned children. That's because sexually abusing children was considered to be normal, acceptable behavior. "Sexual abuse of children was not addressed very openly," wrote one historian, "since taking liberties with a child was often considered merely casual use of an unimportant object."

Infanticide and child abuse were such an accepted part of virtually every culture that they remain the subject of many poems, songs, games, folk tales, and nursery rhymes today. For example, the English version of *London Bridge is Falling Down* tells how iron and lime aren't enough to sustain the bridge. The game, which ends with the capture of another child, is considered an unspoken reference to foundation sacrifices. Indeed, the German version of the song ends with, "All creep through. All creep through. We'll seize the last!"

Hush-a-Bye Baby, probably the best-known lullaby in America, has been called "one of the most blatant infanticide poems." First appearing in 1765 as a Mother Goose Melody, the poem contains children's two most basic fears: loud noises and loss of support.

> *Hush-a-bye, baby, on the tree top*
> *When the wind blows, the cradle will rock;*
> *When the bough breaks the cradle will fall,*
> *Down will come baby, cradle, and all.*

Another poem that is "undoubtedly a relic of something once possessed of an awful significance" is *Ladybird, Ladybird, Fly Away Home.*

> *Ladybird, ladybird,*
> *Fly away home.*
> *Your house is on fire,*
> *And all your children are gone.*

Child murders are also part of popular entertainments. For example, the *Punch and Judy* puppet show has been fascinating children for decades. But behind his colorful clothes, slapstick comedy, and clown-like antics, Mr. Punch has a darker side. Burdened by his marriage and child, Punch wants the freedom to have sex with other women. When Judy finds that Punch has been unfaithful, she flies into a rage, at which point Punch kills her and their child.

Other stories of children at risk aren't hard to find. The *Pied Piper of Hamlin* leads children away from the town, never to return. *The Old Woman in the Shoe* whipped and starved her children. In *Jack and the Beanstalk* the giant threatens, "I'll grind his bones to make my bread." *Tom Thumb*, *The Three Little Pigs*, and *Little Bo-Peep* are all stories of children in jeopardy. And many fairy tales contain witches, giants, bears, and wolves that eat children.

When parents in ancient Rome, Greece, and Persia weren't beating, starving, murdering or sexually abusing their children, they were abandoning them to the elements. Abandonment allowed parents to claim they hadn't committed infanticide, the child's life having been left to the will of the gods.

Abandonment stories were a favorite among the Greeks during the time of Hippocrates—the most famous being that of Oedipus, the son of King Laius and Queen Jocasta. The story begins when an oracle predicts that King Laius will be killed by one of his children. When Oedipus is born, Laius orders his servants to pierce Oedipus's ankles with iron spikes and abandon him on a nearby mountain. (*Oedipus* literally means "swollen foot.") But the servant takes pity on the boy and gives him to a shepherd. Oedipus later fulfills the prophesy by unknowingly killing his father and marrying his mother.

Rome also had its abandonment stories. Numitor, the king of Alba Longa, abandons Romulus and Remus, the mythical founders of Rome, in the river Tiber. A shepherd and his wife later find the twins after they'd been suckled by a she-wolf and fed by a woodpecker.

Indeed, abandonment is the theme of one of the world's most popular folk tales, *Hansel and Gretel*. "Hard by a great forest dwelt a poor woodcutter and his children," it begins. "What's to become of us?" the father laments. "How are we to feed our poor children, when we no longer have anything for ourselves?" "I'll tell you what, husband," says the stepmother. "Early tomorrow morning we will take the children out into the forest to where it is thickest. There we will light a fire for them and give each of them a piece of bread. Then we will go to our work and leave them alone. They will not find the way home, and we shall be rid of them." The wicked stepmother is a favored antagonist in other folk tales, abusing Cinderella and poisoning Snow White.

"The history of childhood," wrote historian Lloyd deMause, "is a nightmare from which we have only recently begun to awaken."

IRONICALLY, WHAT MIGHT HAVE BEEN the single greatest episode of mass infanticide in history spared the child who would later rise up in defense of children.

According to Matthew, in the first century BC, Zoroastrian priests (Magi) warned Herod, king of the Judea Province, that a new king of the Jews had been born. Herod then ordered the Magi to go to Bethlehem and find this newborn king. When the Magi found the boy, they were told by an angel not to tell Herod. *When Herod realized he'd been outwitted by the Magi, he was furious, and he gave orders to kill all the boys in Bethlehem and its vicinity who were two years old and under* (Matthew 2:16).

Later referred to as the Slaughter of the Innocents, Jesus was spared.

CONTRARY TO THE ETHOS of his time, Jesus didn't view children as objects; he believed that anyone who was human couldn't be alien to God, that all were part of God's kingdom. Jesus's love of children is evident throughout the New Testament. For example, He said, *'Suffer little children, and forbid them not to come unto me: for such is the kingdom of heaven'* (Matthew 19:14) and *'whoever welcomes one of these little children in my name welcomes me'* (Mark 9:37). When parents brought their children to Jesus, *He took the children in his arms, placed his hands on them and blessed them* (Mark 10:16).

Jesus's message of love for children was embraced by his followers.

Church fathers argued that children had souls, were important to God, could be taught, and shouldn't be killed, maimed, abused, or abandoned. Indeed, the church was the first institution to provide refuge for abandoned children. Most importantly, the church put pressure on the state to legislate against practices that endangered children, culminating in an historic edict by Constantine, the first Christian emperor of Rome. On May 12, AD 315, state responsibility for the health and welfare of children was born, a direct consequence of the ministry of Jesus Christ. Constantine proclaimed: "Let a law be at once promulgated in all the towns of Italy, to turn parents from using a patricidal hand on their newborn children, and to dispose their hearts to the best sentiments." Religious morality had become state law; infanticide was now a crime. Under the influence of Christian teachings, barbarian tribes also legislated against infanticide.

Then Constantine took Jesus's teachings one step further. In AD 321, he added, "We have learned that the inhabitants of provinces, suffering from scarcity of food, sell and put in pledge their children. We command that those found in this situation . . . be succored by our treasury before they fall under the blows of poverty." This simple directive was the impetus for Christian relief societies for the next eighteen hundred years.

It is hard to overstate the impact of Jesus's teachings on the fate of children. "Amid all the differences of opinion and doctrine that we find among the early founders of Christianity," wrote historian Gregory Henry Payne, "there was one thing on which they were unanimous, and that was the attitude toward children. It was a ceaseless war they waged on behalf of children—those early and oftentimes eloquent founders. From Barnabas, contemporary of the apostles, to Ambrosius and Augustine, they did not cease to denounce those who, no matter what their reasons, exposed or killed infants."

GIVEN JESUS'S LOVE FOR CHILDREN, his support of physicians, and his belief that a God who abhors suffering and comforts the afflicted would never give children diseases as a test of faith, how did we come to a place where parents, in the name of Jesus, are willing to ignore the screams of meningitis, the breathlessness of pneumonia, and the disfiguring erosion of cancer when lifesaving therapies are at hand? The answer lies in the illogical end to a series of events that were first described in the New Testament.

9

THE MIRACLE BUSINESS

"The dearest child of faith is miracle."

—Goethe, *Faust*

Science and religion inhabit two different realms. Science is the study of the natural world; religion is a belief in a world beyond the laws of nature. Science is a matter of evidence; religion, of faith.

For the purpose of this discussion, we're going to make three assumptions:

First: God exists.

Because God isn't bound by the laws of nature, He can do anything, including raise the dead. *At that moment the curtain of the temple was torn in two from top to bottom. The earth shook, the rocks split and the tombs broke open. The bodies of many holy people who had died were raised to life* (Matthew 27:51–52).

Second: Jesus is the Son of God. Because He's the Son of God, He, too, isn't bound by the laws of nature. Jesus could cure leprosy without antibiotics, epilepsy without anti-seizure medicines, and deafness without cochlear implants because He could perform miracles. And, like God, Jesus also brought people back to life: specifically, a widow's son at Nain (Luke 7:11–15); the daughter of a synagogue leader (Luke 8:41–55); and, most famously, Lazarus. *Now a certain man was sick, named Lazarus, of Bethany, the town of Mary and her sister Martha. Then, when Jesus came, he found that he had lain in the grave four days already. Jesus said, 'Take ye away the stone.' Martha, the sister of him that was dead, saith unto him, 'Lord, by this time he stinketh; for he hath been dead four days.' Jesus saith unto her, 'Said I not unto thee that if thou wouldest believe thou shouldest see the glory of God?' And when He thus had spoken, He cried with a loud voice, 'Lazarus, come forth!' And he that was dead came forth'* (John 11:1, 17, 39–44).

IN THE NATURAL WORLD, people who are dead stay dead. That's because of a series of events that occurs seconds after the heart stops beating. Without critical nutrients and oxygen, cells die. As a result, chemical changes in the muscles cause stiffness—called *rigor mortis*—that begins in a few hours and peaks twelve hours later. Also, because the immune system no longer functions, trillions of bacteria that line the nose, throat, skin, and intestines begin to digest the body, producing large quantities of gas that cause massive abdominal bloating. Bacteria also destroy the lining of the nose and palate, causing the brain to slowly seep out. If the person is buried in the earth (like Lazarus), beetles, maggots, insects, and worms consume the muscles. Within a week or so, organs become unrecognizable, melting into a thick, yellow soup.

When Martha said to Jesus that it was too late to resurrect Lazarus because *by this time he stinketh* (John 11:39), she knew what she was talking about. When people die, they produce two foul-smelling organic compounds called *putrescine* and *cadaverine*. Because these substances are part of the natural world, scientists can study them. They can determine their chemical structures; putrescine's is $NH_2(CH_2)_4NH_2$ and cadaverine's is $NH_2(CH_2)_5NH_2$. And they can determine how these compounds act in laboratory cells, in laboratory animals, and in people. Martha's concern that Lazarus had been dead too long was consistent with the laws of nature; her observation that he was successfully brought back to life wasn't. We have to have faith that that's what she really saw.

Some scientists study what happens to people after they die. One is Arpad Vass, an adjunct research professor of forensic anthropology at the University of Tennessee at Knoxville and a senior staff scientist at the nearby Oak Ridge National Laboratory. Vass studies dead bodies after they've been buried in dirt, cement, or seawater. He determines the exact time of death by measuring the quantities of putrescine and cadaverine in various tissue samples. Vass has never found anyone who has come back to life after the heart had stopped beating for more than twenty minutes. Although the resurrections performed by God and Jesus can't be explained by anything that scientists know to be true, it doesn't matter. You either have faith that the dead can be resurrected or you don't.

The third assumption that we're going to make is that mortal men aren't supernatural. Although they might claim to act like God or Jesus, they aren't God or Jesus. So they *are* bound by the laws of nature.

In early Christianity, supernatural acts became the province of mortals at the time of the apostles. *And when Jesus had called unto him his twelve disciples, he gave them power against unclean spirits, to cast them out, and to heal all manner of sickness and all manner of disease* (Matthew 10:1). Jesus commanded the twelve apostles to *'heal the sick, cleanse the lepers, raise the dead, and cast out devils'* (Matthew 10:8). *So they set out and went from village to village, proclaiming the good news and healing people everywhere* (Luke 9:6). Now man, acting as God, had the power to perform miracles. For example, Peter—whose shadow also had miraculous powers (Acts 5:15–16)—cured paralysis (Acts 9:32–35). Philip also cured paralysis (Acts 8:6–7). And Paul, a later apostle, cured snakebites and dysentery (Acts 28:3–9).

The apostles also brought the dead back to life. Peter resurrected a woman in Lydda named Tabitha (Acts 9:36–41) and Paul raised a young man named Eutychus (Acts 20:9–12). Jesus said that anyone who believed in him could perform similar feats. *'Very truly I tell you, whoever believes in me will do the works I have been doing, and they will do even greater things than these'* (John 14:12). No longer were miracles limited to God or Jesus or the apostles; anyone could do them.

As a consequence of these passages in the New Testament, early Christian healing veered in two wildly different directions: one firmly grounded in science; the other, in the supernatural acts of mortal men.

Most impressively, during epidemics, when pagan healers were heading for the hills, Christians rushed into the fray, often risking their lives. Because of their altruism, Christian nurses developed a level of immunity unseen in their pagan counterparts. Christianity won out over paganism because its approach to health, life, and suffering was admirable and persuasive.

But there was another side to Christian healing: a more dangerous side. "A consistent theme in Christianity is to promote direct ministry to the suffering, providing comfort," wrote Richard Sloan in *Blind Faith: The Unholy Alliance of Religion and Medicine.* "This approach encouraged hands-on, practical treatment of disease. At the same time, however, accounts of miraculous healing began to increase substantially. Many of these miracles occurred with the use of relics representing saints and martyrs. Thus, in early Christian times, as in most other eras, the relationship between religion, medicine, and magic was a close one."

Since the first century AD, the Church has been in the miracle healing business.

THE ROMAN CATHOLIC CHURCH boasts more than ten thousand holy men, or saints; many have specific body parts or diseases attached to their names. For example, St. Blaise cures diseases of the throat; St. Appolonia, the teeth; St. Otilia, the head; St. Lawrence, the back; St. Agatha, the breasts; and St. Fiacre, the rectum. In addition, St. Anthony cures *erysipelas* (a skin infection); St. Peregrine, cancer; St. Vitus, epilepsy; and St. Fillan, madness.

The saints didn't have to be alive to work their magic; they could do it with what they left behind: their relics. Many healing orders center on the relics of saints. Christopher Pick, in *Mysteries of the World*, wrote, "Before long, every Christian priest aimed to have a relic of some sort under his church's altar, and with good reason. Whether he liked it or not, a belief in relics and in their alleged power to work miracles formed the core of religion as experienced by the majority of his congregation—many of whom still carried memories of pagan temples and sacred groves in their blood. Holy bones and the like were venerated in every town and village; and, unsurprisingly, a wholesale business in fakes arose to meet this demand."

Relics included the toenails of St. Peter; several heads of John the Baptist; Mary Magdalene's entire skeleton (which included two right feet); scraps of fish left over after feeding the five thousand; a crust of bread from the Last Supper; the arm, two ribs, and the spine of St. Briocus (which apparently "jumped for joy at the honor conferred upon them"); the hand of St. William of Oulx; the fingers of St. Andrew and the Holy Ghost; vials of tears from St. Paul; St. Matthew's arm (which is in the Vatican); the bones of eleven virgin martyrs; the teeth of St. Appolonia; and Lucifer's tail.

The most valued relics were attributed to Jesus, Mary, and Joseph—including Jesus's swaddling clothes, baby hair, baby teeth, and foreskins (sixteen in all); hay from the manger; gifts from the Wise Men; the cloak that Joseph used to cover the infant Jesus; a tear that Jesus shed while resurrecting Lazarus; Jesus's breath in a bottle; His blood; a vessel He used to change water to wine; the tail of the donkey He used to ride into Jerusalem; and the shroud in which He was buried. In addition, churches boast Joseph's staff, hammer, and plows; vials of Mary's breast milk; and rocks onto which her breast milk had fallen. The crucifixion is also well represented—including the entire crown of thorns, nails used to affix Jesus to the cross, and fragments of the cross itself—enough, according to several experts, to build a ship.

Not everyone was comfortable that the Church was in the relics business. In AD 403, Vigilantius of Talouse condemned their veneration as a form of idolatry. But later, Pope Innocent III officially recognized the legitimacy of healing orders centered on relics. He did, however, worry that many relics were forgeries; so, in 1215, he ordered that no one should "presume to announce newly-found relics unless they shall first have been approved by authority of the Roman pontiff." Given that many saints were centuries old, that relics had come from thousands of miles away, and that DNA fingerprinting and carbon dating were still centuries in the future, it's hard to know how the pontiff verified their authenticity.

THE PERFORMANCE OF MIRACLE HEALINGS had extended from God to Jesus to His apostles to saints to martyrs to their relics to priests. It didn't end there. European kings believed that because they ruled by Divine Right, they had a divine ability to heal. Calling it the "royal touch," kings and queens claimed to cure lameness, gout, leprosy, ulcers, and cramps. In 1307, Phillip the Fair, king of France, said he could cure *scrofula* (tuberculosis infection of the lymph glands). Not to be outdone, Charles II, king of England, said he could do it, too, treating five thousand sufferers a year. King Louis XIV of France and the king of Spain also ministered to thousands of sufferers. Although admission was by ticket only, crowds became so large and unruly that people were occasionally killed in the crush. Most kings touched their subjects with coins, rings, or their hands. But not all. King Pyrrhus cured colic by a "laying on of the toes."

BY THE SIXTEENTH CENTURY, one Christian theologian had had enough: Martin Luther, who believed that *only* God and Jesus could perform miracles, not mortal men acting in the name of God or Jesus. He downplayed the physical healings and exorcisms performed by mortals and rejected the superstitions that surrounded saints and their relics. Luther argued that real miracles weren't visible. "Thus Paul says in Romans 8:11 that God will raise up our mortal bodies because of His Spirit which dwells in us," he wrote. "Is this not an immeasurably greater and more glorious work and miracle than if He were in a bodily or temporal way to raise the dead again to life?" In other words, resurrection should be a spiritual, not physical, phenomenon.

Martin Luther influenced Christian philosophy. He did little, however, to change the notion that mortals could act as God, unrestricted by the laws of nature. And so the miracle healings continued—nowhere more so than in a tiny village nestled in the Pyrenees.

AT 12:30 P.M. ON FEBRUARY 11, 1858, an illiterate, asthmatic daughter of a miller in Lourdes, France, had a vision. Bernadette Soubirous, age fourteen, was gathering firewood by the side of a river with her sister and a friend. Suddenly, she heard a noise coming from a hedge and looked up to see "something white" in the form of a young girl about her age. Three days later, Bernadette returned to the grotto with several other girls. While they were kneeling and saying their rosaries, the figure appeared again—but only to Bernadette. Four days after that, on February 18, Bernadette visited the grotto again, this time accompanied by more than a thousand townspeople.

Bernadette stood stiffly, moving her lips while talking to the vision. But again, no one else saw what Bernadette had seen.

It is not clear who later concluded that Bernadette had seen the Virgin Mary. But on March 25, during the Feast of the Annunciation, Bernadette claimed the apparition had said, "I am the Immaculate Conception"—a statement that was both logically and grammatically incorrect. Bernadette's skeptics pointed out that the declaration was more likely the product of an untutored schoolgirl than the voice of the Mother of Jesus. So Bernadette modified her recollection to "I am the Virgin of the Immaculate Conception."

After her vision, Bernadette was rumored to have miraculous powers. She restored the sight of a blind girl by breathing into her eyes and healed a child's paralyzed arm while a dove apparently hovered over her head. Another rumor involved a peasant from the valley of Campan who had doubted Bernadette's apparition; that evening the sins of the doubter were converted to serpents that devoured him without a trace. Another story concerned a moment when Bernadette, while attending sheep, had encountered a rain-swollen stream that parted at her approach. Townspeople treated Bernadette as a saint: "When she left the grotto," recalled one historian, "many people tried to kiss her, and many who could not do so reportedly scraped up earth from her path and kissed this instead. For the masses, Bernadette had become the interpreter if not the image of a superior power."

Bernadette Soubirous created an industry. The Shrine at Lourdes draws about five million visitors a year, claiming thirty thousand healings. Hotel owners and shopkeepers in and around the village enjoy more than four hundred million dollars a year in revenue. Better still, sufferers don't have to travel to Lourdes to be cured. Healing waters obtained from the grotto can be purchased over the Internet for twelve dollars a vial.

Although it's easy to be skeptical about the Shrine at Lourdes, people continue to flock to the site. The reason: they feel better afterwards—much better. In a life drained by misery, sufferers are suddenly the center of attention. "In the Square the sick line up in two rows," wrote one participant. "Every few feet in front of them, kneeling priests with arms outstretched praying earnestly, leading the responses. Nurses and orderlies on their knees are praying, too. Ardor mounts as the Blessed Sacrament approaches. Prayers gather intensity. The Bishop leaves the shelter of the canopy, carrying the monstrance [a vessel in which the consecrated Host is displayed for public adoration]. The great crowd falls to its knees. All arms are outstretched in one vast cry to Heaven. As far as one can see, people are on their knees praying." One pilgrim summed it up best: "Of the uncured none despair. All go away filled with hope and a new feeling of strength. The trip to Lourdes is never made in vain."

BECAUSE OF THE ENORMOUS popularity of faith healing, only two modern-day churches have officially condemned it.

In 1920, the Archbishop of Canterbury, head of the Church of England, concluded, "We can find no evidence that there is any type of illness cured by 'spiritual healing' alone which could not have been cured by medical treatment. The evidence suggests that many such cases claimed to be cured are likely to be either instances of wrong diagnosis, wrong prognosis or spontaneous cure."

In 1962, the United States Lutheran Church Committee agreed with the Church of England, concluding, "Faith healers blame any failure of the healing ceremony on the subject's lack of faith; they ignore any attempt at the use of scientific methodology in their work; the motive is simply a desire for money and the personal power to exploit."

The United Church of Canada came close to rejecting faith healing when, in 1961, it concluded, "Faith healing is not a legitimate ministry of the Church and should be actively discouraged and resisted wherever it is practiced." Six years later, however, the Church relented, claiming there was a difference between authentic faith healing and spurious faith healing.

The only mainstream religious group with an official statement supporting the validity of faith healing is the Roman Catholic Church. In the 1730s, Prospero Lambertini, who would later become Pope Benedict XIV, recognized miracle healings as well as levitations, the duplication of wounds of Jesus's crucifixion, and the spontaneous appearances of Jesus and the Virgin Mary as long as more than one person saw them.

Independent of whether various churches support them, faith healers are here to stay. "The only man with a right to the last word on faith healing," said Reverend George Johnstone Jeffrey, "will be the last man on earth."

Unfortunately, by choosing faith healers, sufferers are relying on mortal men to act as God. And men are fallible, prone to all manner of deceptions. During the past few decades, five Pentecostal ministers have dominated the American faith healing scene.

GRANVILLE "ORAL" ROBERTS was an evangelist-healer who had taken a few theology courses in college. Roberts was the guiding force behind the Oral Roberts Evangelistic Association—a $500-million-a-year enterprise. Headquartered in Tulsa, Oklahoma, Roberts' empire includes Oral Roberts University, the City of Faith Hospital, and the City of Faith Medical and Research Center, all of which attract more than two hundred thousand visitors a year. Roberts claimed to have resurrected "dozens and dozens and dozens" of people during his services. Other claims have been similarly unsupportable. Roberts once brought a California woman onto his show claiming he had cured her cancer; she was dead twelve hours later. That same year, Mary Vonderscher appeared claiming she, too, had been cured of cancer; she was dead three days later. A few years after that, Wanda Beach died after throwing away her insulin at one of Roberts's crusades in Detroit.

PETER POPOFF, "The Anointed Minister of God," was a televangelist in Upland, California, and founder of the Peter Popoff Evangelical Association: an organization that at its peak made more than $4.3 million *a month*. Born in Germany, Popoff claimed he saw his father change water into wine and his mother slice a small piece of bread that fed ten people. Popoff encouraged his audience to throw their medications onto the stage; dozens obeyed, throwing digitalis, insulin, nitroglycerin, and other lifesaving medicines. Popoff also brought his own wheelchairs to revivals and planted healthy people in them, later imploring them to walk: a trick that never failed to stir the audience. James Randi, a professional magician and founder of the James Randi Educational Foundation, later exposed Popoff on the *Tonight Show with Johnny Carson*. Using a computerized scanner during a revival in San Francisco, Randi showed that Popoff had received information about attendees from his wife and members of his staff through a small transmitter in his ear. Randi also planted a man in the audience—dressed as a woman—claiming that he had uterine cancer. Popoff declared that the man's uterine cancer had been cured.

MARION GORDON "Pat" Robertson, a Yale-educated faith healer, is one of the most influential televangelists in the United States. Founder of *The 700 Club* on the Christian Broadcasting Network, Robertson's show, at its peak, was available to more than 80 percent of the American public. Robertson was so powerful that he was considered a viable candidate for president in the mid-1980s. Robertson's healings follow those of many televangelists in that they are broad, poorly defined, and hard to pin down. During one television program, Robertson said, "There is a woman in Kansas City who has sinus. The Lord is drying that up right now. Thank you, Jesus! There is a woman in Cincinnati with cancer of the lymph nodes. I don't know whether it's been diagnosed yet, but you haven't been feeling well, and the Lord is dissolving that cancer right now! There is a lady in Saskatchewan in a wheelchair—curvature of the spine. The Lord is straightening that out right now, and you can stand up and walk." Gerry Straub, a former associate of Robertson's and author of the book *Salvation for Sale*, later wrote, "During my two-and-a-half years at [the Christian Broadcasting Network] I never saw one clear-cut, 'beyond the shadow of a doubt' type of healing; however, I did see a tremendous amount of faith *in* healing—cleverly created, I believe, by Pat Robertson. The prophet-turned-healer could have been described as prophet-turned-fake for the sake of profit."

JIM BAKKER WAS AN Assemblies of God minister and, with his wife Tammy Faye, host of the popular *PTL Club*, which aired on the Christian Broadcasting Network. At their peak, the Bakkers preached to more than twelve million viewers a week. They eventually founded their own television network with weekly contributions of more than one million dollars. "I believe that if Jesus were alive today, he would be on TV," said Bakker. In the early 1980s, the Bakkers built Heritage USA in Fort Mill, South Carolina—at the time, the third most popular theme park in the United States. Between 1984 and 1987, Bakker sold $1,000 lifetime memberships that enabled buyers to spend three days in the luxury hotel at Heritage USA. Bakker raised more than twice the amount of money needed to build the hotel and ended up with far more potential occupants than the hotel could accommodate. Federal officials have a name for this kind of success: fraud. In 1988, after a sixteen-month federal investigation, Jim Bakker was indicted on eight counts of mail fraud, fifteen counts of wire fraud, and one count of conspiracy, having defrauded his flock of $158 million. A jury found him guilty on all counts and sentenced him to forty-five years in federal prison. Bakker also paid $279,000 to Jessica Hahn, a staff secretary at the church, to remain silent about a sexual encounter. In July 1994, Jim Bakker was released from prison after serving five years of his sentence.

JIMMY LEE SWAGGART is a cousin of rock 'n' roll hall of famer Jerry Lee Lewis. Born in Ferriday, Louisiana, and ordained by the Assemblies of God ministry, Swaggart later formed the Family Worship Center in Baton Rouge. At the height of his popularity, Swaggart accused fellow Assemblies of God minister Marvin Gorman of having several affairs. Not to be outdone, Gorman hired his son, Randi, and his son-in-law, Garland Bilbo, to stake out a Travel Inn in New Orleans. The pair took pictures of Swaggart having an affair with a local prostitute named Debra Murphree (who would later appear on the cover of *Playboy*). Gorman tried to bribe Swaggart to recant his accusations against him in exchange for not revealing Swaggart's infidelities. But Swaggart refused, and Gorman went public with what he knew. This led to Swaggart's now famous, "I Have Sinned" broadcast. Elders at the Assemblies of God suspended Swaggart for three months. On October 11, 1991, Swaggart was pulled over by the police in Indio, California, for driving on the wrong side of the road while picking up a prostitute named Rosemary Garcia. "He asked me for sex," Garcia told the patrolman. "I mean, that's why he stopped me. That's what I do. I'm a prostitute." This time Swaggart wasn't contrite, telling his radio and television audience, "The Lord told me it's flat out none of your business." Jimmy Swaggart continues to heal through his radio, television, and Internet broadcasts.

FAITH HEALING HAS BEEN—and will no doubt remain—enormously popular. So if it's all a hoax—run by mortal men with the flaws of mortal men—why haven't people caught on? Two explanations have been offered. One is obvious; the other is harder to admit.

First, faith healers offer a sense of magic and wonder that is lacking in many Christian services. "The most important basis for the growing acceptance of Pentecostal Christianity," writes Tony Campolo, author of *How to Be Pentecostal Without Speaking in Tongues*, "is a hunger in the human psyche for a taste of the miraculous. The truth is that most Christians have a basic dissatisfaction with the quality of their spiritual life and long for something more and something deeper. There is within most of us an insatiable appetite for the supernatural, and mundane Christianity leaves us wanting. We all long for assurances of God's reality in our lives. Rational theologies do not seem to satisfy us, so we look for the ecstasies that are described by the mystics."

The second reason for the enormous popularity of faith healing might be surprising: faith healing works, at least to some extent.

In 2001, Fabrizio Benedetti performed a now classic experiment. He took a blood pressure cuff and put it around the upper arm of volunteers. As the cuff got tighter, subjects experienced greater amounts of pain. As pain increased, volunteers' blood pressure increased, their pulse quickened, they began to sweat, and their muscles contracted. Then Benedetti told volunteers that before he tightened the cuff, he would inject them with morphine, a potent pain reliever. Now, when the blood pressure cuff was tightened, volunteers remained relaxed and pain free.

Next, came the deceit. Benedetti told volunteers that he was going to inject them with morphine when he actually injected them with saltwater (saline). Because saline doesn't relieve pain, Benedetti expected that volunteers would again experience pain as the blood pressure cuff tightened. But they didn't, remaining relaxed and comfortable, just as they had when they'd received the morphine. Benedetti believed he knew why. He reasoned that volunteers had learned to release their own morphine-like drugs called *endorphins*: a contraction of *endo*genous (coming from inside the body) and mo*rphine*. (Endorphins are made in parts of the brain called the *pituitary* and *hypothalamus*.) To prove his theory, he injected Naloxone instead of saline. Naloxone blocks the effects of endorphins. As predicted, volunteers again experienced intense pain. What this study proved was that people could *learn* to produce their own pain-relieving chemicals. Studies like those of Benedetti haven't been limited to pain relief. For example, patients with Parkinson's disease can learn to release their own dopamine, which alleviates symptoms. And some people can learn to enhance or suppress their own immune systems. So it's possible that *believing* you are being healed causes the body to undergo physiological changes that promote healing.

Another way that faith healing might work is that people think they're better when they're not. One study performed at Harvard Medical School showed how this was possible. Ted Kaptchuk and coworkers studied forty-six patients with asthma. To some he gave albuterol (a bronchodilator that helps relieve the symptoms of asthma), and to others he gave saline. Then Kaptchuk asked patients to breathe out as hard as they could until it felt like no air was left in their lungs; this is called forced expiratory volume, or FEV. Kaptchuk found that patients who received albuterol had a 20 percent increase in FEV while those who had received saline had only a trivial increase. Most interesting was how patients *thought* they did. About 50 percent of subjects in both groups thought they had improved, even though only the albuterol group actually had.

The most dramatic example of how expectation determines outcome is the now-famous sham surgery study. In 2002, Nelda Wray and coworkers at Baylor College of Medicine studied 180 patients with arthritis of the knee. Some had arthroscopic surgery to remove loose cartilage, and others had sham surgery in which an incision was made but nothing was done. Patients didn't know which of the two surgeries had been performed. Remarkably, both groups claimed success, experiencing less pain and better mobility following the surgery. *Thinking* you had knee surgery was as good as *having* knee surgery.

Improvement in symptoms caused by saline or sham surgery is called a placebo response. As a general rule, the Food and Drug Administration (FDA) won't license drugs, biologicals, or vaccines until they're compared with placebos and shown to be better. However, just because something doesn't work *better* than a placebo doesn't mean that it can't work *as* a placebo. Indeed, much of faith healing is based on the power of the placebo response. Expectation is everything.

UNFORTUNATELY, THE PLACEBO response can only do so much. So, when parents choose their faith over lifesaving medical therapies or lifesaving vaccines for their children, they have crossed an important line. Children can't make decisions for themselves. They depend on their parents to protect them; and if their parents put them in harm's way, they depend on others to step in. Sadly, others almost never do.

10

THE PECULIAR PEOPLE

"The First Amendment embraces two concepts—freedom
to believe and freedom to act. The first is absolute. The
second cannot be."

—OWEN ROBERTS, ASSOCIATE JUSTICE,
UNITED STATES SUPREME COURT

Although the choice to withhold lifesaving medical therapies
from children in the name of religion is surprising, more surprising is that citizens, lawmakers, and prosecutors haven't stepped
forward to stop it. It wasn't always that way. Beginning more than
a hundred years ago, the law consistently protected children against
religiously motivated medical neglect.

It started with the Peculiar People.

IN THE MID-1800s, John Banyard founded the Peculiar People. Located in Essex, England, the Peculiars took their name from 1 Peter
2:9, which calls the Lord's followers *a royal priesthood, a holy nation,
a peculiar people*. Like all faith healers, the Peculiar People rejected
modern medicine, choosing prayer and anointment instead.

In 1868, Lois Wagstaffe, the fourteen-month-old daughter of
Mary Ann and Thomas Wagstaffe, died of pneumonia. Believing she
was suffering from teething, the Wagstaffes called on church elders

to anoint her with oil. After Lois died, the Wagstaffes were charged with manslaughter because, as noted by a local official, "it was lamentable to think that there should be such a perversion of Scripture with respect to children."

The law, however, was on the Wagstaffes' side. According to British common law, "in the absence of a statute declaring it a positive duty upon a parent to call in a medical practitioner, the omission to do so can scarcely be considered negligence so gross and wanton as to be criminal." After the Wagstaffes were acquitted, several jurors publicly decried the absence of a law to protect children from medical neglect. Their pleas reached the British Parliament. Six months later, the Poor Law Amendment Act was modified to read, "when any parent shall willfully neglect to provide adequate food, clothing, *medical aid*, or lodging for his child . . . whereby the health of such child shall have been injured . . . [the parent] shall be guilty of an offense." The state now had a right to prosecute parents who medically neglected their children.

The first test of the new law came in 1875 when a Peculiar named John Robert Downs chose prayer to treat his thirteen-month-old daughter's scarlet fever. After she died, Downs was charged with manslaughter, convicted, and sentenced to three months in prison. Downs's imprisonment didn't change behavior; the Peculiar People continued to deny their children medical care.

In 1882, British citizens saw just how devastating the Peculiar People's actions could be. During the trial of John and Rachel Morby—whose eight-year-old son, Abraham, had died from smallpox—Rachel explained that she, her husband, and their other children had been "out and about" during their son's fatal illness. Her admission was in direct violation of smallpox quarantine laws. At the inquest, the coroner asked, "Do you think your creed authorizes you to murder a street full of people?" The jury convicted John Morby of manslaughter.

The most sensational trial of the Peculiar People occurred in 1897 when George Senior's fourteen-month-old son, Amos, contracted pneumonia. Senior chose prayer and anointment, without success. It wasn't the first time that a child of George Senior's had died. It was the sixth. "The Lord gave and the Lord hath taken away," he explained. Senior was convicted of manslaughter. Then, on December 15, 1898—five days after the court upheld his conviction—Senior's eight-month-old son, Tansley, died of pneumonia. Confronted with the fact that Senior had now lost seven of his twelve children to illness, the judge sentenced him to four months in prison with hard labor.

The Downs, Morby, and Senior cases opened a floodgate of convictions. During the second half of the nineteenth century, Peculiars were charged, convicted, and imprisoned when their children died from diphtheria, epilepsy, and a variety of other illnesses.

British courts had spoken. Parents who chose to medically neglect their children in the name of God could be convicted of a crime and sent to prison. The most amazing aspect of the British cases wasn't *that* they occurred but *when* they occurred. The Peculiar People were successfully convicted of letting their children die from diphtheria before diphtheria antiserum, from seizures before phenobarbital, and from pneumonia and scarlet fever before antibiotics.

The final and most influential trial of the Peculiars occurred in the early 1920s after Norman Purkiss, the three-year-old son of Louisa and Henry Purkiss, died of diphtheria. The difference between the Purkiss case and the others was that it occurred *after* diphtheria antiserum had become available. The prosecutor pointed out that parents were "perfectly entitled" to anoint themselves with oil when they were sick, but they weren't entitled to do the same to their sick children. Two decades later, these words would echo almost verbatim in what would become the single most cited public health case ever argued before the United States Supreme Court.

EVENTS IN THE UNITED STATES soon mirrored those in England.

In the spring of 1901, Emma Judd and her newborn "were lulled into eternity by the prayers of John Alexander Dowie"—a leader of a faith healing sect in Chicago—after they failed to receive medical care during a complicated childbirth. Chicago's citizens were in an uproar, fueled in large part by the unrepentant arrogance of both Dowie and Emma's husband, John. Unfortunately, John Dowie hadn't broken any laws. A local newspaper wrote, "The general opinion among lawyers [is] that the laws as presently shaped are inadequate to cope with this modern evil."

The Judd case in America paralleled the Wagstaffe case in England. Soon prosecutors, judges, and child advocates targeted Dowie and his followers, eager to prevent them from causing more harm. The most famous politician to rise in defense of children was presidential hopeful William Jennings Bryan, who said, "There should be a limit to so-called religious freedom. And the limit should be reached when folly usurps the throne of the Christian faith." Bryan's anger was ironic, given his fervent defense of the Bible during the "trial of the century," in which John Scopes was accused of teaching evolution in violation of Tennessee state law—a trial that was later immortalized in the play and movie *Inherit the Wind*.

As had been the case in England, public outcry changed the law. The first test came one year after the death of Emma Judd and her baby.

In 1902, Luther Pierson, a clerk for the New York Central Railroad, chose prayer instead of medical care for his daughter's pneumonia. Pierson was a member of the Christian Catholic Church, a faith healing group. "All diseases are the devil," he said, "and it was the devil's work in this child." Pierson was confident that "the Almighty would arrest disease if I asked him." When his daughter died, Pierson blamed himself: "I attribute the child's death to a lack of faith on my part, and to the fact that I am not pure in the sight of

God." In May 1901, a White Plains, New York, jury found Pierson guilty of criminal neglect. Pierson later took his case to the New York State Court of Appeals, which supported the conviction, writing that Pierson "cannot be excused from punishment for slaying those who had been born to him."

The Pierson case showed that parents in the United States who chose prayer instead of medicine could be convicted of a crime and sent to prison. "The verdict is of the highest importance," said J. Addison Young, a Westchester County district attorney, "and means absolutely that these faith curists and others of the same sort must obey the law." An editorial in the journal, *American Lawyer*, hailed the verdict as a blow "to all members of the great cult of humbuggery."

ALTHOUGH THE PIERSON VERDICT was important, the final word on religiously motivated medical neglect won't be made by local courts, district courts, or state courts; it will be made by the United States Supreme Court. Unfortunately, Supreme Court justices have never ruled on a faith healing case. They have, however, handed down verdicts in many cases involving the First Amendment guarantee to practice religion freely and without restraint. Eight cases have been particularly instructive. The driving principle behind these decisions seems to be that if a religious practice doesn't hurt society, it's permitted; if it could hurt society, it's not.

IN FOUR CASES, Supreme Court justices have not allowed states to regulate religious practices.

In 1963, Adell Sherbert, a Seventh-day Adventist living in South Carolina, was fired from her job as a textile worker. Like all Adventists, Adell didn't work on Saturdays: a practice inspired by Exodus 20:10: *The seventh day is the Sabbath of the Lord thy God; in it you shalt not do any work.* Two years after Adell had joined the church, her employer switched from a five-day to a six-day work week, including Saturdays. Because Adell couldn't work and maintain her faith at the same time, she quit. When she couldn't find other work, she applied for unemployment compensation, which was denied. The South Carolina Employment Compensation Commission argued that because Adell had quit, she wasn't entitled to anything. So she took her case to the South Carolina Supreme Court—and lost. The case then went to the United States Supreme Court which, by a vote of 7 to 2, struck down the previous decision, agreeing with Adell that her First Amendment right to practice religion freely had been violated.

IN THE LATE 1960s, Jonas Yoder, Wallace Miller, and Adin Yutzy—Amish parents living in New Glarus, Wisconsin—took their children out of school after the eighth grade, believing that sending them to a local high school would endanger their salvation. Everything their children needed to know, they argued, could be learned on the farm. Their choice, however, was in direct violation of a Wisconsin state law requiring children to attend school until they were sixteen. The case worked its way up to the United States Supreme Court, where justices sided with the parents. But not all were comfortable with the decision. Justice William O. Douglas, worried that his fellow justices had opened a dangerous door, sounded a note of caution: "The power of the parent, even when linked to the free exercise claim of the first amendment, may be subject to limitation *if it appears that parental decisions will jeopardize the health or safety of the child.*"

IN 2005, AN UNUSUAL alliance between the George W. Bush administration, liberal activists, and conservative religious groups rose in support of five Ohio prisoners who had been prohibited from conducting religious services. Two prisoners were followers of Asatru, a polytheistic Viking religion that reveres Thor; one was a minister of the Church of Jesus Christ Christian, which preaches white supremacy; the fourth was a Wiccan witch; and the last was a Satanist. The United States Supreme Court voted unanimously to support the prisoners' right to practice their faith unimpeded by the Ohio state correctional system.

PERHAPS THE MOST INTERESTING clash between religious freedom and societal norms took place in Hialeah, Florida, in the late 1980s. In 1954, Ernesto Pichardo arrived in South Florida with the first wave of Cuban exiles, settling in an area of Miami called Little Havana. Ernesto embraced his mother's belief in Lukumi-Santeria, an ancient religion rooted in Yorubaland, West Africa. Yorubas worship *orishas*, guardians of human destiny. It was how they worship them that became the problem.

Yorubas believe that in order to remain strong and effective, *orishas* must eat; otherwise, human lives are in jeopardy. Nothing apparently nourishes *orishas* better than animal blood. As a consequence, the Santerian calendar is a smorgasbord of animal sacrifices including chickens, goats, roosters, pigeons, ducks, turtles, hens, doves, lambs, rams, and rats. After the sacrifice, animals are eaten according to the saying, *"La sangre para el Santo, la carne para el Santero"* ("Blood for the Saint, meat for the Santerian").

By the 1980s, more than fifty thousand Santerians lived in South Florida. In 1987, responding to the growing need for a place of worship, Ernesto Pichardo opened the Church of the Lukumi Babalu Aye in an abandoned car dealership two blocks from Hialeah's main street and city hall.

Unfortunately for Pichardo, at the time he opened his church, several sensational events involving Santerians had alarmed the American public. In nearby Miami, worshippers had placed animal carcasses on the steps of courthouses—offerings they hoped would bring good luck to those on trial. In New York City, goats' heads and paper bags filled with bloodied chicken feet appeared in Central Park. In Falls Church, Virginia, police found gutted chickens in a local cemetery. And in Santa Monica, California, pools of blood were found in a parking lot following the ritual sacrifice of three lambs. The religious practices of Santerians further frightened the public when a popular television show, *Miami Vice*—based on two real-life Miami-Dade detectives—featured haunting episodes about Santeria worshippers. And in 1987, the movie *The Believers*, starring Jimmy Smits, Helen Shaver, and Martin Sheen, implied that Santerian sacrifices weren't limited to animals.

As tensions built, Santerians found themselves in court in violation of recently passed health ordinances. The *Miami Herald, Washington Post, New York Times*, and *Los Angeles Times* called them "the chicken wars." It wasn't long before Ernesto Pichardo's church in Hialeah was at the center of the controversy.

The city of Hialeah—perhaps best known for a racetrack that features four hundred pink flamingos—consists mostly of Cuban Americans living in small houses and apartments. Confronted with Pichardo's new church, neighbors got together to shut it down. The lawyer they hired was Alden Tarte. "Santeria is not a religion," said Tarte. "It is a throwback to the dark ages. It is a cannibalistic, Voodoo-like sect, which attracts the worst elements of society: people who mutilate animals in a crude and most inhumane manner. Ernesto Pichardo is not the kind of guy you want next door." Pichardo disagreed. "It's just a continuing process of religious persecution," he said. Pichardo didn't have the resources to fight his neighbors. But help was at hand. The Miami chapter of the ACLU agreed to take the case.

On October 5, 1989, Pichardo lost in federal court. Judge Eugene Spellman ruled that "Santeria remains an underground religion and the practice was not, and is not today, socially accepted by the Cuban population." Spellman estimated that "between twelve thousand and eighteen thousand animals are sacrificed in initiation practices alone." Pichardo's lawyer, Jorge Duarte, was appalled by the verdict. "It is a dark day for religious freedom," he said. "We've made criminals out of seventy thousand people in South Florida." Next, Pichardo appealed Spellman's verdict to the Eleventh Circuit's Court of Appeals. Again, no luck. In a tersely worded, one-paragraph opinion, the court upheld Spellman's verdict. But Pichardo wasn't finished. On March 23, 1992, the United States Supreme Court agreed to hear the case.

Fifteen months later, Supreme Court justices handed down their ruling. Writing for the majority, Justice Anthony Kennedy chastised city officials for using sanitation ordinances to harass Pichardo's church. "Our review confirms that the laws in question were enacted by officials who did not understand, failed to perceive, or chose to ignore the fact that their official actions violated the nation's essential commitment to religious freedom." Ernesto Pichardo had won his fight to practice his religion freely. On learning of the decision, Pichardo held a news conference. "This is why we came to the United States," he said, "because we have freedom of speech and freedom of religion. Animal sacrifice is an integral part of our faith. It is like our holy meal." Evoking the name of the *orisha* of thunder and lightning, Pichardo said, "Shango was on our side."

Two weeks after the verdict, Rigoberto Zamora, a Pichardo supporter, celebrated by performing a public sacrifice. "What before we had to hide," he said, "now we can do in the open." With cameras rolling, Zamora sacrificed a ram, three goats, five chickens, two roosters, two pigeons, and two guinea hens. Then he poured the ram's blood over an altar dedicated to Shango. "We feel different now," he enthused, "but we have always done this, legal or not." Unfortunately, the two-hour ceremony didn't go quite as planned. Because he had used a dull steak knife, Zamora had trouble severing the head of the ram. And he had to kill one of the guinea hens by slamming its head against the floor. Then he ripped off the head of a pigeon with his hands. Media coverage wasn't kind.

ACCORDING TO THE United States Supreme Court, states do not have the right to limit the religious practices of employees who can't work on the Sabbath; of parents who choose to home school their children; of prisoners whose religious beliefs include witchcraft, white supremacy, reverence to Thor, and allegiance to Satan; and of people who want to offer the blood of freshly sacrificed animals to appease holy spirits.

IN FOUR INSTANCES, however, Supreme Court justices have allowed states to regulate certain religious rituals.

In the history of public health, no case has been cited more than that which began one night on the streets of Brockton, Massachusetts. In the early 1940s, Sarah Prince, a Jehovah's Witness, asked her niece, Betty Simmons, to help distribute pamphlets in exchange for voluntary contributions. Betty wasn't coerced to hand out the reading materials; in fact, she enjoyed it. Unfortunately, Betty's pamphleteering was in direct violation of a Massachusetts child-labor law that prohibited boys under twelve and girls under eighteen from "selling, exposing, or offering for sale any newspapers, magazines, periodicals or any other articles of merchandise of any description in any street or public place." The purpose of the statute was to keep children out of potentially dangerous situations. Sarah Prince was convicted of violating this law. Eventually, she took her case to the United States Supreme Court.

During the trial, Prince argued that her niece was exercising her "God-given right and her constitutional right to preach the gospel." The Court disagreed. In a strongly worded verdict, Justice Wiley B. Rutledge wrote, "The family itself is not beyond regulation in the public interest. And neither the rights of religion nor the rights of parenthood are beyond limitation." Then, echoing the words of the prosecutor in the case of Peculiar Norman Purkiss, Rutledge wrote, "Parents may be free to make martyrs of themselves, but they are not free in identical circumstances to make martyrs of their children."

THE SECOND INSTANCE in which the Supreme Court ruled against religious practices was the first case to set limits on the First Amendment. It occurred almost a hundred years before Sarah Prince distributed her religious pamphlets on the streets of Brockton.

In the 1860s, George Reynolds married Amelia Jane Schofield—which wouldn't have been a problem if he hadn't still been married to Mary Ann Tuddenham: a fact he didn't deny. Reynolds, a member of the Church of Latter-day Saints, was arrested for polygamy.

In the early 1800s, no religious group was more vilified than the Mormons. Persecuted in New York and in other East Coast cities, they fled to the Midwest where their founder, Joseph Smith, further inflamed the public by introducing the doctrine of polygamy, which Smith believed paved the way to heaven. To escape further persecution, Smith's successor, Brigham Young, continued the Mormon migration westward, ending up at the Great Salt Lake Basin in Utah. In 1852, polygamy was officially embraced as a church doctrine. In response, the United States Congress passed a series of statutes forbidding polygamists to serve on juries or vote in federal elections. But Mormons refused to give in. So, in 1862, Congress made polygamy a crime, passing the Morrill Anti-Bigamy Act. During deliberations, Congress relied on the words of Thomas Jefferson who, in his Bill for Establishing Religious Freedom, wrote, "the acts of the body, unlike the operations of the mind, are subject to coercion of the laws." In other words, people can believe whatever they want; they just can't do whatever they want.

On October 23, 1874, a grand jury indicted George Reynolds for polygamy. A few months later, Reynolds was convicted and sentenced to two years of hard labor and ordered to pay a five-hundred-dollar fine. Reynolds, refusing to believe he had done anything wrong, took his case to the United States Supreme Court.

In 1878, Supreme Court justices handed down their ruling. Chief Justice Morrison Waite stated, "To permit [polygamy] would be to make the professed doctrines of religious belief superior to the law of the land, and in effect to permit every citizen to become a law unto himself." Under such circumstances, argued Waite, government would exist in name only. Then Waite went even further, taking the plea for religious freedom to its illogical end. "Suppose one believed that human sacrifices were a necessary part of religious worship," he wrote, "would it be seriously contended that the civil government under which he lived could not interfere to prevent a sacrifice? Or if a wife religiously believed that it was her duty to burn herself upon the funeral pile of her dead husband, would it be beyond the power of the civil government to prevent her from carrying her belief into practice?"

George Q. Cannon, a Mormon and a representative of the Utah territory, was angered by the Court's ruling, saying, "Our crime has been that we married women instead of seducing them; we reared children instead of destroying them; and we desired to exclude from the land prostitution, bastardy, and infanticide. If George Reynolds is to be punished, let the world know that in this land of liberty the law is swiftly invoked to punish religion, but justice goes limping and blindfolded in pursuit of crime."

THE THIRD INSTANCE in which the Supreme Court allowed states to regulate religious practices occurred in the 1980s. This time, the Court ruled on a religious ritual that violated state drug laws.

Alfred Smith and Galen Black were counselors at a private, non-profit alcoholism and drug treatment center in Roseburg, Oregon. As a condition of employment, all counselors were asked to refrain from "any and all alcoholic beverages and other mind-altering substances unless prescribed by a physician."

Smith and Galen were members of the Native American Church, which uses peyote as part of its religious ceremony to "communicate with the Creator and obtain spiritual enlightenment." Peyote contains the powerful hallucinogen mescalin: a Schedule I drug in the same class as heroin, cocaine, and marijuana. In Oregon, as in many states, the use of Schedule I drugs is a criminal offense. When Smith and Galen were found to have used peyote during a religious ceremony, they were fired from their jobs. When they applied for unemployment insurance, their claims were denied.

The case eventually worked its way up to the United States Supreme Court. Lawyers for Smith and Galen argued that peyote didn't hurt anyone; that other Schedule I drugs such as marijuana were legal in some states; that illegal trafficking of peyote didn't exist; and that the use of peyote was an act of worship, similar to the ingestion of wine during communion. Lawyers for the state argued that allowing peyote for religious purposes would make it difficult to enforce existing drug laws, burden the criminal justice system, and allow for religious claims for the use of other psychedelic drugs such as LSD, hashish, and heroin. "State criminal law would become a patchwork of prohibition," they argued, "covering some people for some drugs, and other people for other drugs."

Smith and Galen lost their case. Writing for the majority, Justice Antonin Scalia agreed with the Employment Division of Oregon, arguing that the Supreme Court had never held that an individual's religious beliefs should excuse him from compliance with valid drug laws.

THE FOURTH SUPREME COURT case limiting religious practice was probably the most heart wrenching. The issue at hand, however, was so clear that justices didn't bother to write a lengthy opinion.

In 1945, following the widespread use of blood transfusions in World War II, Jehovah's Witnesses officially condemned the practice, likening it to "cannibalism." Their position ignited a series of high-profile court cases.

In 1952, an infant named Cheryl Linn Labrenz suffered from a disorder that destroyed her red blood cells. Without a blood transfusion, she would surely die. Her mother, a Jehovah's Witness, argued that the transfusion "would be breaking God's commandment." A judge in Cook County, Illinois, appointed a guardian to take over Cheryl's care and ordered him to consent to a blood transfusion. The Illinois State Supreme Court upheld the ruling.

In 1961, a three-year-old boy named Joseph Perricone suffered a heart condition that required an immediate blood transfusion. His father, a Jehovah's Witness minister, argued that it violated Biblical scripture. The judge disagreed. Unfortunately, by the time Joseph had received the transfusion, he was too ill to benefit, dying fifteen minutes later. A jury later convicted the Perricones of child neglect. The New Jersey State Supreme Court upheld the conviction.

In 2004, twin sons of Jehovah's Witnesses Jason and Rebecca Soto suffered a disorder called twin-twin transfusion, when one twin inadvertently transfers much of his blood to the other while still in the womb. As a consequence, the twin who loses blood can became severely anemic. Jason and Rebecca, however, refused a transfusion for their son. The hospital sought and received a court order for temporary custody of both children. The lower court granted the request, and the Nevada State Supreme Court upheld it.

Laws requiring blood transfusions have also extended to children before they're born. In 1964, a hospital in Neptune, New Jersey, sought a court order to transfuse a woman named Willimina Anderson who suffered from a disorder in which the placenta blocks the exit of the child from the womb. If left unattended, the blockage can cause massive hemorrhaging during the birth process, killing both mother and child. Willimina, a Jehovah's Witness, refused the transfusion. In this case, Willimina wasn't making a decision for herself only. The New Jersey State Supreme Court granted the order, stating that it was "satisfied that the unborn child is entitled to the law's protection." Willimina's husband disagreed. "Our religion calls for man to do God's will," he said, "yet six men on the Supreme Court of New Jersey have overruled God's will."

Perhaps the most unusual case of Jehovah's Witnesses involved Jesse E. Jones. One evening, Jones, who suffered from a bleeding ulcer, was taken to a Washington, DC, hospital after she had lost a lot of blood. Her husband refused to allow her to receive the blood transfusion needed to save her life. The hospital sought a court order mandating the transfusion. Judge J. Skelley Wright agreed, and Jesse's life was saved. Unique to this case, Judge Wright appears to have countermanded the Supreme Court's ruling in the case of Sarah Prince, which stated, "Parents may be free to make martyrs of themselves . . ." Jesse Jones was prepared to martyr herself only; unlike Willimina Anderson, she wasn't pregnant. She was, however, the mother of a seven-month-old child. The judge ruled that, "The state will not allow a parent to abandon a child, and so it should not allow this most ultimate of abandonments."

Eventually, the United States Supreme Court weighed in. In 1968, in response to a Washington State Supreme Court ruling that centered on a little boy severely injured in an automobile accident, the justices supported the lower court's ruling ordering blood transfusions for the children of Jehovah's Witnesses. The case was so clear that the justices didn't write a single sentence in support of their opinion, choosing instead to write one word: *affirmed*.

In four instances, United States Supreme Court justices have ruled that certain religious practices—because they might be detrimental to society—can be regulated by the state. Specifically, states can prevent young children from standing on street corners at night;

compel children of Jehovah's Witnesses to receive lifesaving blood transfusions; prohibit polygamy and its potential for debasement of women and children; and ban the use of a powerful hallucinogen. Although faith healing cases have never come before the United States Supreme Court, one can only imagine that justices would similarly rule that denying children lifesaving medicines is also contrary to the good of society.

THEN, ON JUNE 30, 2014—in what Justice Ruth Bader Ginsburg called "a decision of startling breadth"—the United States Supreme Court broke new ground.

Several years earlier, President Barack Obama introduced the Affordable Care Act, which required all corporations employing more than fifty people to provide minimum essential health coverage, including contraception. Two companies, Hobby Lobby, a chain of craft stores, and Conestoga Wood Specialties, a manufacturer of wood cabinets, balked. While company owners were willing to provide coverage for condoms, diaphragms, sponges, birth control pills, and sterilization surgery, they were unwilling to provide intrauterine devices (IUDs) and morning-after pills, which, because they induce abortions, violate their Christian values.

Before the Hobby Lobby decision, the Supreme Court had considered the religious rights of individuals and religious groups; now, for the first time in history, it was considering the rights of for-profit corporations acting as religious groups. By a vote of five to four, the Supreme Court sided with company owners, arguing that they didn't have to provide contraception services if they held a "sincere religious belief" that doing so would be wrong.

In a scathing dissent, Ginsburg argued that the Court had just "ventured into a minefield." Company owners could now impose their religious beliefs on employees who didn't necessarily share those beliefs. What if companies run by Jehovah's Witnesses refused coverage for blood transfusions; or Scientologists refused antidepressants; or Muslims, Jews, or Hindus refused medical products containing porcine gelatin, such as anesthetics, intravenous fluids, or pills; or Christian Scientists refused vaccines; or Catholics refused AIDS medications or services for same-sex couples? "The court forgets that religious organizations exist to serve a community of believers," wrote Ginsburg. "For-profit corporations do not fit that bill."

The Obama administration was similarly appalled. Josh Earnest, the White House press secretary, said "women should make personal health decisions for themselves, rather than their bosses deciding for them."

Two other aspects of the Hobby Lobby decision were particularly unsettling. First, the Court had ignored the science. Although executives at Hobby Lobby and Conestoga Wood Specialties had argued that IUDs and the Plan B morning-after pill induce abortions, they don't. According to research at the Mayo Clinic, National Institutes of Health, and other academic centers, both of these contraceptive devices prevent fertilization, not implantation. Second, and perhaps most disturbing, was the fact that five men on the United States Supreme Court had made a decision for the nation's women. Dorit Reiss, a professor at the University of California Hastings School of Law, summed it up best. "It's hard to read this as anything but gendered," she wrote. "Our monotheistic religions are all the products of times when the equality of women was not at the forefront."

DESPITE THE LACK OF a specific Supreme Court ruling on faith healing, parents in the United States—beginning in the early 1900s—have been consistently charged, convicted, and sentenced to prison for medically neglecting their children in the name of God. In the mid-1970s, however, the clarity provided by these earlier rulings began to unravel. As a consequence, district attorneys in most states now have a hard time prosecuting parents.

The confusion occurred during the Nixon administration—at a time, ironically, when Americans were most interested in putting an end to child abuse.

11

THE DIVINE WHISPER

"To cure is the voice of the past.
To prevent, the divine whisper of today."

—*British Medical Journal*, 1903

In the summer of 1874, a woman lay dying of tuberculosis on the top floor of a tenement building in New York City. A Methodist missionary found her there and asked if she could help. "My time is short," said the sick woman, "but I cannot die in peace while the miserable little girl whom they call Mary Ellen is being beaten day and night by her stepmother next door."

Mary Ellen lived in the home of Francis and Mary Connolly, though she wasn't a blood relative of either. She was the illegitimate daughter of Mary's late first husband, Thomas McCormick. The Methodist missionary's name was Etta Angell Wheeler. When Wheeler entered the Connolly's apartment, she found Mary Ellen thinly dressed, barefoot, and bruised. "She was a tiny mite," said Wheeler, "the size of five years, though she was nine. She struggled [to wash] a frying pan about as heavy as herself. Across the table lay a brutal whip of twisted leather strands and the child's meager arms and legs bore many marks of its use. I went away determined, with the help of kind Providence, to rescue her from her miserable life."

It wasn't going to be easy. First, Wheeler went to the police. "Unless you can prove that an offense has been committed," they said, "we cannot interfere. And all you know is hearsay." Next, Wheeler went to the administrators of several benevolent societies. Again, she was rebuffed. "If the child is legally brought to us, and is a proper subject, we will take it," they said, "otherwise, we cannot act in this matter." But Wheeler wasn't giving up. "I will make one more effort to save this child," she said. "There is one man in this city who has never turned a deaf ear to the cry of the helpless. I will go to Henry Bergh."

In 1866, eight years before Etta Wheeler walked into his office, Henry Bergh founded the Society for the Prevention of Cruelty to Animals. Wheeler reasoned that, at the very least, children were part of the animal kingdom. Bergh listened to Wheeler's story. "If there is no justice for her as a human being," he said, "she shall at least have the rights of the stray cur on the street." Bergh's first act was to find justice for Mary Ellen.

The trial was a media sensation. Among the first to testify was Mary Ellen herself. "I have no recollection of ever having been kissed by anyone," she said. "I have never been kissed by my mamma. I have never been taken on my mamma's lap and caressed or petted. I have never dared to speak to anybody, because if I did I would get whipped." Jacob Riis, a police reporter, described the scene. "I was in a courtroom full of men with pale stern looks," he wrote. "I saw a child brought in, carried in a horse blanket, at the sight of which men wept aloud. I saw it laid at the feet of the judge, who turned his face away, and in the stillness of that courtroom I heard a voice raised claiming for [Mary Ellen] the protection men had denied her. The story of little Mary Ellen stirred the soul of the city and roused the conscience of the world that had forgotten. And, as I looked, I knew I was where the first chapter of children's rights was written."

The case of Mary Ellen dominated New York City newspapers for months. When it was over, Mary Connolly was sentenced to a year in prison; Etta Wheeler took custody of Mary Ellen; and Henry Bergh founded the Society for the Prevention of Cruelty to Children, the first organization of its kind. Its mission was clear: "To convince those who cruelly ill-treat and shamefully neglect little children that the time has passed when this can be done with impunity."

During the next twenty years, the Society investigated more than a hundred thousand cases of suspected child abuse. As described by Charles Flato in *The Saturday Evening Post*, the stories were grim: "Children have been whipped, beaten, starved, drowned, smashed against walls and floors, held in ice water baths, exposed to extremes of outdoor temperatures, and burned with hot irons and steam pipes. Children have been tied and kept in upright positions for long periods. They have been systematically exposed to electric shock; forced to swallow pepper, soil, feces, urine, vinegar, alcohol, and other odious materials; buried alive; had scalding water poured over their genitals; had their limbs held in open fire; placed in roadways where automobiles would run over them; placed on roofs and fire escapes in such a manner as to fall off; bitten, knifed, and shot; and had their eyes gouged out. The reports of injuries read like the case book of a concentration camp doctor." Within a few decades of its founding, the Society for the Prevention of Cruelty to Children had successfully prosecuted twenty-one thousand offenders and rescued more than thirty thousand children.

It was just the beginning.

In the 1930s, one medical invention proved that child abuse was far more common than anyone had realized: X-rays. Sadly, it took radiologists years to understand what they were looking at. When they did, Americans understood for the first time the magnitude of the epidemic around them—and supported legislation to prevent it.

In 1945, John Caffey, a radiologist at the College of Physicians and Surgeons at Columbia University, published a paper in the *American Journal of Roentgenology*. Caffey described four children with "thickenings in several bones." All four were less than three months old. "[These patients] suffered from none of the recognized conditions in which thickenings had been found previously, such as scurvy, rickets, syphilis, bacterial osteitis [bone infection], neoplastic disease [cancer], or traumatic injury." The thickenings were a mystery. "After prolonged investigation of four patients," wrote Caffey, "the cause remained undetermined. Traumatic injury was not observed in a single case either at home or in the hospital."

The following year, Caffey published another paper in the same journal, reporting six more children with bone thickening. This time the thickenings, now believed to be fractures, were accompanied by subdural hematomas: collections of blood between the skull and the brain. "Some of the fractures in the long bones," wrote Caffey, "were caused by the same traumatic forces which were presumably responsible for the subdural hematomas." Again, parents appeared baffled. Caffey noted that these children were frequently bruised; were pale and malnourished; and always got better in the hospital and worse after they left. One child in the report returned after only a few days with five new fractures around the knee. For the first time, Caffey considered that parents might be hiding something. "In one of the cases," he wrote, "the infant was clearly unwanted by both parents, and this raised the question of intentional ill-treatment." Still, Caffey was hesitant to take the next step, hesitant to accuse parents of intentionally hurting their children. "The evidence was inadequate to prove or disprove this point," he wrote, meekly.

In 1956, ten years after John Caffey had made his observations, Fred Silverman published a paper titled "The Roentgen [X-Ray] Manifestations of Unrecognized Skeletal Trauma." Unlike Caffey, Silverman was willing to point a finger at abusive parents: "It is not often appreciated that many individuals responsible for the care of infants and children may permit trauma and be unaware of it, may recognize trauma but forget or be reluctant to admit it, *or may deliberately injure the child and deny it.*"

The tipping point came six years later.

In 1962, Henry Kempe published a paper titled "The Battered Child Syndrome." This time the manuscript wasn't published in a specialty journal for radiologists; it was published in the *Journal of the American Medical Association*, the most widely read medical journal in the world. "The battered child syndrome," wrote Kempe, "is a frequent cause of permanent injury or death. The syndrome should be considered in any child exhibiting evidence of fracture in any bone, subdural hematoma, failure to thrive, soft tissue swellings, or skin bruising, in any child who dies suddenly, or where the degree and type of injury is at variance with the history given regarding the occurrence of the trauma." Kempe reported 750 children with X-ray evidence of past abuse. Seventy-eight had died. One hundred fourteen had suffered permanent brain damage.

Unlike the papers of Caffey and Silverman, Kempe's was accompanied by a press release. Within a few weeks, *Time, Newsweek, Life, The Saturday Evening Post*, and every major newspaper in the country were writing about child abuse. One article was titled, "Parents Who Beat Children: A Tragic Increase in Cases of Child Abuse Is Prompting a Hunt for Ways to Select Sick Adults Who Commit Such Crimes." During the next twenty years, medical journals published more than seventeen hundred articles about child abuse. By the mid-1970s, child abuse had its own medical journal; Henry Kempe was the editor.

KEMPE'S ARTICLE—and the media attention that followed—opened the eyes of a nation. X-rays no longer allowed parents to deny that they'd been serially abusing their children. Congress took notice. In

1971, presidential hopeful Senator Walter Mondale (D-Minnesota) created the Senate Subcommittee on Children and Youth, a power base from which he would mobilize Congress to protect children. In 1972, the subcommittee published a book titled "Rights of Children," setting the stage for Mondale's seminal piece of legislation: the Child Abuse Protection and Treatment Act (CAPTA).

At 9:30 A.M. on March 26, 1973, in the wood-paneled offices of the Dirksen Senate Office Building, Walter Mondale opened the hearings. It was the first time in history that Congress had addressed the issue of child abuse. The second person to testify was the most riveting: a woman identified only as Jolly K.

> MONDALE: Did you abuse your child?
>
> JOLLY K: Yes, I did, to the point of almost causing death several times.
>
> MONDALE: I don't want to embarrass you, but can you tell me what happened?
>
> JOLLY K: It was extreme serious physical abuse the two times. Once I threw a rather large kitchen knife at her and another time I strangled her because she lied to me.
>
> MONDALE: How old was the child?
>
> JOLLY K: Six-and-a-half-years old.
>
> MONDALE: And did you have repeated examples of abuse?
>
> JOLLY K: Yes. It was ongoing. It was continuous. These were not isolated instances. With parents who have this as an ongoing problem it is the difference between getting drunk on New Year's Eve and getting drunk every day.

Jolly K. explained that she had beaten her daughter in much the same manner as she had been beaten as a child. She hadn't, however, told her whole story; a story that included a childhood of abandonment, rape, foster homes, juvenile halls, and repeated delinquency;

and a womanhood of prostitution, bad marriages, and attempted suicide. Toward the end of her testimony, Jolly K. described how she had founded Parents Anonymous, a support group for parents who abused their children. At the time of Mondale's hearings, Parents Anonymous had helped more than four thousand families.

Although he had frequently butted heads with Richard Nixon, Mondale eventually got the legislation he wanted. "Not even Richard Nixon is in favor of child abuse!" he quipped. Mondale's bill allocated $86 million for a center within the Department of Health, Education, and Welfare (now the Department of Health and Human Services) that would compile a list of accidents involving children, publish training materials for case workers, and create a national commission to study the effectiveness of state surveillance. By the mid-1970s, all fifty states had mandatory child-abuse-reporting laws.

The impact was immediate. In 1963, public authorities had identified more than a hundred thousand cases of child abuse; by 1982, the number had climbed to 1.3 million. Advocates hailed the new legislation as a watershed event for children's rights. But not everyone was celebrating. One group saw the legislation as a direct threat to its way of life. And it was going to do everything it could to exempt itself from public scrutiny.

IN 1967, FIVE-YEAR-OLD Lisa Sheridan had a cough, fever, and difficulty breathing. Suffering from bacterial pneumonia, she could have been cured with antibiotics. Her mother, Dorothy, a Christian Scientist, chose prayer instead. At autopsy, more than a quart of pus was found in Lisa's chest, collapsing her right lung and pushing her liver downward. The Massachusetts district attorney charged Dorothy Sheridan with involuntary manslaughter. Although Dorothy was remorseless, the child's grandmother was appalled. "How could a mother let a sweet, dear child die of neglect," she said, "when the laws of our land make us pick up a dog hurt in an accident and take it to the nearest veterinarian?" Dorothy Sheridan was sentenced to five years of probation. Elders in the Christian Science Church saw the trial of Dorothy Sheridan as a wake-up call; if she could be prosecuted for following the tenets of her faith, all of them were at risk. CAPTA was about to shine an unwanted light on their way of life. Something had to be done. So church authorities turned to the two men they were certain could help.

ON JUNE 17, 1972, five men broke into the headquarters of the Democratic National Committee in the Watergate office complex in Washington, DC. A few days later, President Richard Nixon ordered his chief-of-staff, H. R. "Bob" Haldeman, to instruct the CIA to block the FBI's investigation into the source of funding for the burglars. It didn't work. Investigators soon traced cash and checks in the burglars' possession to a fund dedicated to Nixon's reelection campaign. As investigations intensified, John Ehrlichman, Nixon's chief advisor for domestic affairs, misinformed the Attorney General that no one in Nixon's White House had any prior knowledge of the burglary. When the dust settled, forty-eight government officials were found guilty of perjury, conspiracy, and obstruction of justice: many were sent to prison. Although Nixon was never indicted, he faced almost certain impeachment; so he resigned from office, later to be pardoned by Gerald Ford.

Haldeman and Ehrlichman shared several features: both were lawyers; both were powerful men in Nixon's White House; both were of German descent (dubbed by the press "the Berlin Wall" for their fierce protection of the president); both were heavily involved in the cover-up that led to Nixon's resignation; both were indicted, convicted, and jailed for their crimes; and both were Christian Scientists. Although the Watergate scandal consumed much of their efforts from June 1972 until their resignations on April 30, 1973,

Haldeman and Ehrlichman still had enough time to insert a religious exemption into CAPTA: "No parent or guardian who in good faith is providing a child treatment solely by spiritual means—such as prayer—according to the tenets and practices of a recognized church through a duly accredited practitioner shall for that reason alone be considered to have neglected the child."

Haldeman and Ehrlichman had tipped their hand; only Christian Scientists would refer to their prayers as *treatments* and to faith healers as *practitioners*; and only the Christian Science Church *accredits* its healers.

Now, if state officials didn't abide by Haldeman and Ehrlichman's mandate, they couldn't receive money from Mondale's program; within a few years, forty-nine states (the exception being Nebraska) and the District of Columbia had laws protecting religiously motivated medical neglect. By 1984, the Department of Health and Human Services, realizing the absurdity of the mandate, eliminated it. But it was too late. The damage had been done.

NO CASE BETTER ILLUSTRATES the confusion created by CAPTA than that of Amy Hermanson.

On September 30, 1986, Amy Hermanson, the seven-year-old daughter of Christian Science parents, died of untreated diabetes. Insulin would have saved her life, but her parents chose prayer instead. Six days before Amy died, her mother, Christine, took her to a piano lesson for one of her adult students. Midway through the lesson, Amy crawled up to her mother and begged to be taken home. The student, frightened by Amy's appearance, urged Christine to call a doctor; but she refused, saying, "She'll be alright." On the last day of her life, Amy lay in bed vomiting and urinating uncontrollably, attended by her parents, a Christian Science nurse, and a member of the Christian Science Committee for Publication, who forbade the nurse from calling 9-1-1. In 1989, the Hermansons were charged and convicted of felony child abuse and third-degree murder. At the time of the trial—and as a direct result of Haldeman and Ehrlichman's additions to CAPTA—Florida had a religious exemption to civil charges for child abuse (a misdemeanor, which typically results in a fine or community service) but not for criminal charges (such as manslaughter, felony child endangerment, or murder, which typically result in imprisonment). In other words, a choice to medically neglect a child for religious reasons couldn't be a civil offense but could be a criminal offense. This apparent contradiction was confusing for both parents and prosecutors.

In 1992, the Florida Supreme Court overturned the Hermansons' convictions. Judges argued that religious exemption laws failed to clearly spell out the parents' obligations: "A person of ordinary intelligence cannot be expected to understand the extent to which reliance on spiritual healing is permitted and the point at which this reliance constitutes a criminal offense. The statutes have created a trap that the legislature should address." In other words, it shouldn't be left to parents in Florida to figure out when they had crossed the line from a civil to a criminal act.

The problem created by Haldeman and Ehrlichman continues. As of 2013, thirty-eight states and the District of Columbia still had religious exemptions for child abuse in their civil codes, and seventeen had religious exemptions for felony crimes. In the end, these ambiguities benefit no one. Not children, who may be denied life-saving therapies. Not parents, who remain uncertain about when the line is crossed to criminal behavior. Not prosecutors, who are often unclear about what constitutes medical neglect. And not society, which is charged with protecting its youngest, most vulnerable members. The issue won't be resolved until all fifty states eliminate religious exemptions from both civil and criminal child abuse statutes.

PERHAPS WORST OF ALL, the courts have often failed to protect children at risk *before* they've been harmed. One recent example of this took place on a small farm outside of Cleveland, Ohio.

In May 2013, ten-year-old Sarah Hershberger was diagnosed with an aggressive form of lymphoma at Akron Children's Hospital. Her parents, Anna and Andy Hershberger, who are Amish, live and work on a farm in Medina County, Ohio, about thirty-five miles southwest of Cleveland. Doctors at the hospital explained that with chemotherapy, Sarah had an 85 percent chance of survival. But it wasn't going to be easy; chemotherapy has side effects, often causing nausea, vomiting, lack of energy, and loss of hair. The Hershbergers agreed to the chemotherapy, and Sarah's tumors started to shrink. But the treatment took a toll. "It put her down for two days," said Andy. "She was not like her normal self. We just thought we cannot do this to her." Instead, the Hershbergers, after "seeking the wisdom of God," discontinued the chemotherapy and treated Sarah with herbs and vitamins instead. When told that Sarah could die within a year, Andy Hershberger said that he was willing to take that chance.

In response to the Hershbergers' decision, Maria Schimer, a nurse and lawyer for Akron Children's Hospital, sought limited guardianship of Sarah, hoping to complete the course of chemotherapy that would likely save her life. But the Hershbergers refused. On July 31, the case went before Medina County Judge John Lohn, who sided with the parents, making statements that were arguably irrelevant, illogical, and at variance with the United States Constitution.

First: Lohn stated that the Hershbergers were "good parents," a fact that was irrelevant to the case. It didn't matter whether Sarah's parents were attentive or neglectful. In either case, they shouldn't have had the right to decide whether Sarah lived or died when a life-saving therapy was at hand.

Second: Lohn argued that Sarah had "begged her parents to stop the treatments" because they made her feel sick. No ten-year-old wants chemotherapy; side effects occur in almost everyone who receives them. But serious diseases require serious medicines. While herbs and vitamins were surely more tolerable, they also wouldn't treat her disease.

Third: Lohn said that "there is no guarantee that chemotherapy would be successful." This is true for all medical therapies. For example, children with bacterial meningitis receive antibiotics that dramatically lessen but don't eliminate the chance of being permanently harmed or killed by the disease. The lack of a 100-percent guarantee doesn't mean that parents could reasonably choose not to treat meningitis. Similarly, chemotherapy, which offered Sarah an 85 percent chance of survival, was clearly better than herbs and vitamins, which offered her a 0 percent chance of survival.

Finally, and most depressingly, Lohn wrote that "there was no law and no basis in fact for [Akron Children's Hospital] to file this action." However, there might well have been a "basis in fact" for Akron Children's Hospital to do what it had done. Because, despite the confusion created by CAPTA, there's a way out of this.

THE MOMENT WHEN *all* American children should have been legally sheltered from the abuses of their parents occurred on July 9, 1868, with the passage of the Fourteenth Amendment. The Equal Protection clause of that amendment is clear: no state shall "deny to any person within its jurisdiction the *equal protection of the laws*." In other words, children aren't entitled to less protection under the law simply because their parents hold a certain religious belief—even those whose devoted parents wrongly believe, after seeking God's wisdom, that herbs and vitamins can cure cancer. When justices of the United States Supreme Court ruled that creating separate schools for African American and white children was unconstitutional, lawyers cited the Fourteenth Amendment's Equal Protection clause (*Brown v. the Board of Education of Topeka, Kansas*). Later, the Equal Protection clause opened the door to integration in all aspects of American life. Because of the Fourteenth Amendment, courts have struck down laws discriminating against children with severe developmental delays as well as those born of illegal immigrants or born out of wedlock.

Probably the clearest opinion that rested on the Equal Protection clause occurred in the Ohio Court of Common Pleas in 1984. The case involved a thirteen-month-old boy named Seth Miskimens, who died after his parents chose prayer instead of antibiotics when pus filled the sac around his heart (pericarditis), making it virtually impossible for his heart to expand and contract. The Court upheld the conviction of the parents with a ruling that should have been a death knell to all religious exemptions to medical care for children: "Why should children not be afforded special protection by our laws, each child on an equal basis with every other child, where the denial of that protection may injure or cripple the child for life or even result in the child's premature death? *Equal protection should not be denied to innocent babies, whether under the label of 'religious freedom' or otherwise.*"

Akron Children's Hospital appealed Lohn's decision. On August 27, 2013, the appeals court sided with the hospital, noting that the child also had rights. Maria Schimer, the lawyer representing the hospital, was thrilled. "We believe this case is about children's rights," she said, "and about giving a ten-year-old girl an 85 percent chance of survival."

Schimer's joy was short-lived.

When the appeals court ruled in favor of the hospital, a taxi was sent to the Hershberger's home. But no one was there, the family having gone into hiding. On February 14, 2014, Maria Schimer dropped the case, claiming "it was impossible to make medical decisions for the child after she went into hiding." By dropping the case, Schimer had effectively allowed the Hershbergers to return to their farm after a four-month absence. An attorney for the Hershbergers hailed the decision as "a small win for parental rights." In all likelihood, however, it will be a major loss for Sarah.

In the case of Sarah Hershberger—as is true in virtually all faith healing cases—the parents do all the talking. And what they talk about is their religious freedoms. But this isn't about the rights of the parents; it's about the rights of the child. The fact that Christian Scientists and other faith healing groups have successfully made these cases an issue of their First Amendment right to religious freedom rather than their children's right to have a life has been a triumph of misdirection. "If they can get you asking the wrong question," wrote Thomas Pynchon in *Gravity's Rainbow*, "they don't have to worry about the answers."

On November 12, 1993, Bob Haldeman died of abdominal cancer at his home in Santa Barbara, California; true to his beliefs, he had refused all medical treatments. On February 14, 1999, John Ehrlichman died from complications of diabetes in Atlanta; unlike Haldeman, Ehrlichman had left the Christian Science Church, choosing dialysis to treat his kidney failure. Ironic, given that he had almost single-handedly created a loophole that has allowed parents to legally deny such lifesaving measures to their children.

12

STANDING UP

"Evil thrives when good men do nothing."

—EDMUND BURKE,
IRISH STATESMAN AND AUTHOR

One woman, however, has made it her life's mission to undo what Bob Haldeman and John Ehrlichman had done. After her son died, Rita Swan wanted to learn more about the child with meningitis who had recovered completely with prayer: a boy named Danny, whom the Christian Science Church had been touting as another faith healing success. Why had prayer worked for Danny but not for her son? What had she done wrong? "I had to know whether that was true," recalled Rita. "So I called the church in that town and a week later the boy's mother called me back. Her little boy was seventeen years old. Because his dad was not a Christian Scientist, he eventually insisted that the boy get medical care. He was diagnosed with viral meningitis. I thanked her for sharing her story and hung up, but was confused. She made no mention of antibiotics yet doctors had told us antibiotics were the necessary treatment."

So Rita visited the Wayne State University Medical Library and read about the different types of meningitis. "For me, the most liberating moment was when I was reading textbooks in the medical library," said Rita. "I could just barely understand any of it. But I did understand that the boy with viral meningitis had a different disease. Matthew had bacterial meningitis. He needed antibiotics." (Matthew Swan had died from meningitis caused by *Haemophilus influenzae* type b [Hib]: a bacterial infection that could have been treated with antibiotics, and for which a vaccine became available ten years later. Danny, on the other hand, had suffered from viral meningitis, which typically resolves on its own, antibiotics being both useless and unnecessary.) "News of Danny's recovery had been spread through the church as proof that Christian Science could have healed Matthew, but the comparison was [inaccurate]," recalled Rita. "I was so relieved that I sat on the floor of the library stacks reading the section over and over. I did not have to be afraid that Matthew had died because we were not right with God. I didn't have to be afraid of leaving Christian Science. I knew that I wasn't giving up a magical, supernatural protection or any kind of protection from evil because Christian Science had no power. It hadn't healed anything."

ON JANUARY 1, 1979, Rita Swan decided to tell her story to the world: "I said to myself that I am going to try to do something every day to bring this issue to the attention of the public." First, Swan wrote a forty-nine-page manuscript that she hoped would be published, at least in part, by a local newspaper. "All through 1979 I tried to find print media that would be interested but it was just too strong for them. They didn't want to publish a blistering attack on Christian Science." Both her local Grosse Pointe paper and the *Detroit Free Press* turned her down. So did several magazines. No one was willing to take on Christian Science. "I think that the *Christian Science Monitor* had too much prestige in the print media world," she observed.

Next, Swan called the executive producers of the most popular talk show in America: *The Phil Donohue Show*. In November 1979,

Donohue opened his show to stunned silence from his studio audience. "The Swans are here to tell a very complicated and very painful story," he began. "Their fifteen-month-old son died. And it is their belief that he died because they formally subscribed to the principles of Christian Scientists. Obviously they are very bitter, confused, angry, and resentful." Then, taking off his glasses and looking directly into the camera, Donohue paused dramatically: "Before we begin: one announcement. A sincere effort was made to engage a representative of the Christian Science Church. And although three representatives flew in from headquarters in Boston and spent an hour with our associate producer, they declined to appear on the program."

The Swans then did something that had never been done before. In front of millions of television viewers, they lay bare a major established religion. "We were not casual Christian Scientists," said Doug Swan. "We were officers in the church. We were Sunday school teachers. We were on boards of the church. We had published in Christian Science magazines. We knew what the Church taught." Rita then explained how they had come to appear on the show: "There is nothing that would have driven us out of the Church if we hadn't seen an innocent child killed in that way. He trusted us." Later, she referred to her former religion as "a fragile magic."

The response to the show was immediate. "We got about six hundred letters," recalled Rita. "Many from ex-Christian Scientists who were amazed that this kind of thing would see the light of day." Amazed that anyone would dare to take on a religious belief, even one that meant occasionally sacrificing children to the false notion that prayer alone heals. And the letters kept coming.

When Rita and Doug Swan appeared on *The Phil Donohue Show*, they were the first Christian Scientists to openly oppose the Church on national television. Ten years later, when they appeared on *Donohue* again, nothing had changed. "We're still the only former Christian Scientists in the country who will talk about this," said Rita. "We've lost virtually every Christian Science friend we ever had."

IN 1983, FIVE YEARS after Matthew's death, the Swans founded Children's Healthcare Is a Legal Duty (CHILD), one of the most successful child advocacy organizations in the United States. "We do not believe that society should have allowed us to do what we did to our child," said Rita. First, Rita wanted to shine a light on those who, like her, had medically neglected their children in the name of God. She wanted the press and the public to see the silent epidemic around them. So she teamed with Seth Asser, a pediatrician from San Antonio, Texas, and combed the nation. On April 4, 1998, in an article titled "Child Fatalities from Religion-Motivated Medical Neglect," they published their findings in *Pediatrics*, the official journal of the American Academy of Pediatrics.

Swan and Asser had examined newspaper articles, trial records, personal communications, public documents, police records, coroners' files, and other confidential materials—finding 172 children who had died under suspicious circumstances during the previous twenty years. They found a two-year-old boy whose treatable kidney tumor weighed six pounds and a twelve-year-old girl whose bone cancer was the size of a watermelon. They found a two-year-old girl who had accidentally inhaled a small piece of a banana, in response to which her parents called a special prayer meeting while she struggled to breathe, turned blue, and died in front of them. They found a twenty-three-year-old woman who had come to an emergency room after fifty-six hours of active labor because her baby's head was stuck at the vaginal opening. The dead baby, delivered by caesarian section, "was in an advanced stage of decomposition." The mother died within hours from puerperal sepsis: a bloodstream infection. The coroner noted that "the corpse of the infant was so foul smelling that it was inconceivable that anyone attending the delivery could not have noticed." Another medical examiner commented on the mother's death: "That's an infection that doesn't even occur today. You read about it in the textbooks from the 1910s—the pre-antibiotic era."

Swan and Asser also found children who had died from treatable bacterial infections such as pneumonia, meningitis, and sepsis. A one-year-old girl named Eva Swanson died of sepsis after she had accidentally spilled a pot of scalding tea on herself. A fifteen-month-old boy named Dustin Gilmore "was deafened, blinded and killed" by meningitis. In each case, the parents never looked back, never questioned their choice to put their faith in God rather than in doctors. One mother, who had lost her baby to pneumonia, said, "Jesus was the doctor."

At the time the article appeared, no one really knew how frequently medical neglect in the name of God was occurring in the United States. Swan and Asser's report offered the first glimpse. The authors found twenty-three denominations in thirty-four states that practice faith healing; tens of thousands of Americans were refusing medical care for themselves and their children. Five sects accounted for most of the deaths: Christian Science, Church of the First Born, End Time Ministries, Faith Assembly, and Faith Tabernacle. In discussing their findings, the authors made an ominous projection: "We suspect that many more fatalities have occurred during the study period than the cases reported here." Swan and Asser knew that deaths in faith healing sects were often reported as due to natural causes. And they knew that many deaths were never reported. They feared they had seen only the tip of the iceberg. And they were certain the abuse was continuing. It was like "watching Jonestown in slow motion," said Asser.

A few months after Asser and Swan's article was published, a gravesite was discovered outside Oregon City, Oregon. It belonged to an insular group called the Followers of Christ Church. Investigators found seventy-eight children buried there: almost half had died before their first birthday. None had been included in Asser and Swan's report. To observers, the cemetery looked like it had been transported from the sixteenth century into the twentieth. According to investigators, the Followers have witnessed more childhood deaths than any other religious sect in modern times.

Swan and Asser also knew that, for every death, hundreds of other children were suffering or permanently disabled. Such as children who developed hearing loss from untreated ear infections, or paralysis from untreated bacterial meningitis, or heart valve defects from untreated strep throats, or chronic kidney disease from untreated urinary tract infections, or shortened limbs from unhealed fractures, or blindness from untreated diabetes, or brain damage from complicated home deliveries. And then there are all the children who have to suffer frequent seizures from untreated epilepsy or breathing attacks from untreated asthma.

To put these stories in perspective, every year in the United States, a bacterium called *meningococcus* causes about five hundred cases of bloodstream infections and meningitis in children. No bacterium spreads fear in the community more quickly than this one; children are often fine one minute and dead four hours later. Although antibiotics are available to treat meningococcus, the disease's onset is so rapid and overwhelming that by the time the child gets to a hospital, it's often too late. Investigators at the CDC say they can determine the incidence of meningococcal infections by simply reading about cases in local newspapers. What most people don't realize is that far more children suffer every year from religion-inspired medical neglect than from meningococcus. Meningococcal disease can largely be prevented by spending hundreds of millions of dollars every year vaccinating teenagers; religiously motivated medical neglect can be prevented by simply changing the law.

Since she founded CHILD, Rita Swan has presented at fifty conferences and symposia, appeared on forty-five local and national television programs, written thirty articles and editorials in newspapers and magazines, testified before twenty-four local, state, and federal legislative hearings, and written one book, *The Last Strawberry*, which describes in painful detail the story of her son, Matthew. As a direct result of her lobbying efforts, several advocacy groups have issued strongly worded statements against religious exemptions from child abuse and neglect laws: specifically, the American Academy of Pediatrics, the United Methodist Church, the American Medical Association, the National District Attorneys Association, the Massachusetts Citizens for Children, Prevent Child Abuse America, and the National Association of Medical Examiners. And five states have completely eliminated religious exemptions from child abuse laws: Oregon, Hawaii, Massachusetts, Maryland, and North Carolina.

Some have argued that Rita Swan is wasting her time—that even if religiously motivated parents know their actions could land them in jail, they will still continue to do what they're doing. Continue to see God, not man, as the ultimate authority. One prosecutor lamented how hard it would be to get a conviction even if the law was on his side: "You bring in these parents, sobbing and upset that their child died, and they say that is what God told them to do. If they truly believe that and a jury believes they are sincere, you are not going to convict them of any crime." Further, the courts have historically never punished those whom they considered to be unalterably delusional, unable to tell the difference between right and wrong. Sigmund Freud, who considered religious zealotry to be a form of mental illness, supported this position.

Swan's efforts, however, have proven to be anything but a waste of time. The threat of jail, as it turns out, has been quite an effective deterrent.

Punishment for breaking the law serves two purposes. The first is retribution. People are punished to make them suffer as they had made others suffer. The second is utilitarian. People are punished as a warning to others who might consider committing similar crimes. It's the difference between punishing a child and punishing him in front of his brothers and sisters. The child is punished so that he will not do something wrong again; the child is punished in front of his siblings so that they won't do something wrong. Criminals are punished today so that there will be less crime tomorrow. The question for those who choose prayer instead of medicine is: Would punishing those who choose to medically neglect their children in the name of God prevent them from doing it again? Or prevent others from doing it? Several recent events have provided an answer.

The Christian Science Church teaches its members that religious exemptions to medical neglect exist because legislators know that prayer can be as effective as standard medical treatments. If state legislators changed the law, they would be sending a message that prayer is not an acceptable replacement for good medical care. "Christian Scientists are law-abiding people," said Rita Swan. "We were very submissive that way. If we knew it was the law, we did it. For example, we got our dog rabies shots. If we had known it was the law to get our child medical care, we would have been relieved to do that." David Twitchell, a Christian Scientist who had chosen prayer instead of surgery for his son's bowel obstruction, later remarked that had he known he could have been prosecuted, he would have done it differently. "I don't know what I was thinking," he said.

In Canada and Great Britain, where religious exemptions don't exist, faith healers must seek conventional therapies for children who are ill—if they don't, they can be charged with a crime. In Canada, two children have died from faith healing, in Great Britain, none.

Perhaps no state has shown how changing the law can change behavior more than Oregon. "The Oregon story is incredibly powerful," said Rita Swan. "For decades, children died in this one church—the Followers of Christ Church—and nobody cared. The coroner didn't care. The prosecutor didn't care. Nobody paid any attention. And the deaths continued."

Then one prosecutor decided to swim upstream, to confront the reluctance of people in his state to challenge the totality of religious freedom. "In 1998, I spoke at a National Child Abuse Conference," recalled Rita, "and a prosecutor from Oregon ran up to me afterwards and said we've got a lot of these deaths in my county and I'm a new prosecutor and I really want to do something about it." The new prosecutor's name was Terry Gustafson. Three weeks after Rita spoke at the conference, an eleven-year-old boy from the Followers of Christ Church in Oregon died of untreated diabetes.

"By 1997, Oregon had religious defenses to murder by abuse or neglect, manslaughter, criminal mistreatment, criminal non-support, failure to provide, and neglect," recalled Rita, all the direct result of Christian Science lobbying. Gustafson knew she couldn't file any charges until the laws were changed. "Well, I can't file charges," she said, "but at least I can go to the press." So she went to the press, and the press went to the cemetery of the Followers of Christ Church and found seventy-eight young children buried there. Investigators discovered eighteen children who had died in the past ten years; three had died in the previous seven months—all could have been saved. One child, a six-year-old named Holland Cunningham, died after two-thirds of his bowel got stuck in a hernia. The local coroner described the pain that would have accompanied his death as "unimaginable." Then the press went to a satellite congregation in Idaho and found the graves of twelve more children.

Now the public was on board. In 1999, Representative Bruce Starr introduced a bill that repealed all religious exemptions in Oregon. "Then the Christian Scientists entered," recalled Rita, "well-dressed professionals who constantly besieged legislators. So what do legislators do when two groups take strong, passionate, opposing positions on a bill? Split the difference!" Legislators ended up repealing five of the exemptions. It wasn't perfect. But at least it provided a large enough window for prosecutors to file charges. Because of mandatory sentencing guidelines, Oregon parents who are convicted of child abuse or neglect could spend as much as twenty-five years in jail. After the bill was signed into law, Starr's office was flooded with phone calls from members of the Followers of Christ Church asking what they needed to do to stay within the bounds of the law. In the eighteen months before the law was changed, three children among the Followers died. In the nine years after the law was changed, one child died. "We hoped that the compromise bill would be enough to persuade the Followers to change their behavior," recalled Rita, "and for many years it seemed that it had. But in 2008 and 2009, three Followers' children died without medical care, and in 2010 a fourth was permanently harmed by medical neglect."

Again, Rita Swan stepped forward. "In 2010, I contacted Bruce Starr and asked if he would be willing to [seek] repeal [of] the other religious exemptions. He said that he would." So Rita and Doug Swan moved to Oregon to fight the fight worth fighting. "We found a college student to live in our Iowa home, bought studded snow tires for crossing the Rockies, boxed up 250 pounds of stuff to ship by truck, and loaded the rest of our necessities in the car, leaving our Labrador retriever, Boomer, just enough room to lie down in the back seat. We lived in Salem for four months." Their efforts paid off. "To our surprise, the Christian Science Church quickly gave up," said Rita. "The Church sent a letter to legislators saying it would not oppose the bill because the deaths of children in Oregon were 'tragic' and have, and I quote, 'reached critical mass.' When we lobbied for repeal of these religious exemptions in 1999, when there were seventy-eight children buried in the Followers of Christ cemetery, the Christian Science Church fought us tooth and nail. But in

2011, when there were eighty-three children buried there, the deaths had reached critical mass." An irony that wasn't lost on either Swan or the legislators.

In June 2011, the governor of Oregon signed the bill into law. Religious exemptions to civil or criminal charges have now been completely eliminated. And there hasn't been a single death of a child among the Followers of Christ Church in Oregon since. "We have evidence . . . that many members of the Church are now quietly taking their children to doctors," said a local district attorney. "We're very hopeful in the long term that we won't have to prosecute these cases anymore."

Following Oregon's change in the law, several members of the Followers of Christ Church moved to Idaho, which has a religious exemption to manslaughter and where the death rate among the children of the Followers is ten times greater than in the general population. Swan will consider her mission complete when every state in the union stands up for the right of children to have a life. But it's not going to be easy. Rita Swan's success in Oregon was followed by a stunning defeat in Pennsylvania. A defeat made all the more surprising in that it followed a case of pedophilia that drew international media attention.

THE STORY READS like a biblical parable.

In November 2011, Penn State University was immersed in scandal. A Centre County, Pennsylvania, grand jury had charged Jerry Sandusky with molesting eight boys during the previous fifteen years. Sandusky was a former assistant Penn State football coach, the founder of a charity for troubled children, and a beloved member of the Penn State community. No one could believe it. But the boys—most of whom were now men in their 20s—told the same story. Sandusky had plied them with computers, golf clubs, tickets to football games, and, most seductively, a chance to have the father figure they all so desperately needed. After he had gained their trust, he sodomized them, either in the basement of his house or in the locker room showers on campus.

What people couldn't understand was how he'd gotten away with it. Surely someone must have known about this. As it turns out, they did. One, Jim Calhoun, a locker room attendant at Penn State, reported what he'd seen to his supervisor. "I fought in the Korean War," said Calhoun. "[I've seen] people with their guts blowed out and arms dismembered. [But] I just witnessed something I'll never forget." Calhoun didn't report what he'd seen to the police. Neither did his supervisor. Another assistant Penn State football coach, Mike McQueary, a former quarterback for the team, had also heard Sandusky raping a young boy in the shower. He told Penn State's head coach, Joe Paterno, who told the athletic director, Timothy Curley. McQueary also reported what he'd seen to Penn State's vice president, Gary Schultz, who informed Graham Spanier, Penn State's president. Again, no one did anything. They didn't call the police, and they didn't try to find the boy. It was as if—similar to the Book of Job—the Devil had made a bet with God. The Devil would put an evil man in a community full of good men and wait to see who would be the first to stand up. No one did. So the abuse continued.

Finally, someone had the courage to come forward. But it wasn't any of the adults in supervisory positions; it was one of the victims. Identified as Victim Number One, he had repeatedly been molested between 2007 and 2008. In June 2012, a jury found Jerry Sandusky guilty on forty-five counts of sexual assault. Sandusky will spend the rest of his life in jail. His victims will spend the rest of theirs dealing with the trauma.

THE JERRY SANDUSKY scandal at Penn State University generated a public outcry for stronger laws and stiffer penalties against child abuse. The result was Pennsylvania Senate Bills 20 and 28. First introduced in March 2013, the bills made it clear that child abuse was a crime that would not be tolerated. Now, by law, adults in Pennsylvania will have committed a crime if they "cause serious bodily injury" by "kicking, biting, stabbing, cutting, or throwing a child" or "unreasonably confine or restrain a child" or "forcefully shake or slap a child under one year of age" or "cause a child to be near a methamphetamine lab" or "operate a vehicle in which a child is a passenger while driving under the influence of alcohol or a controlled substance." Indeed, parents could be convicted of a crime even if there was only "*reason to believe* that a child was endangered."

ON THURSDAY, APRIL 13, 2013, while Pennsylvania Senate bills 20 and 28 were being debated, Brandon Schaible, the seven-month-old son of Herbert and Catherine Schaible, died. For several days, Brandon had suffered difficulty breathing, diarrhea, constant crying, and fitful sleep. The Schaibles prayed, but to no avail. The Philadelphia coroner pronounced the child dead at 8:35 P.M.

To the Schaibles, this was familiar territory.

Three years earlier, in 2009, Herbert and Catherine Schaible chose prayer instead of antibiotics for their two-year-old son, Kent, when he contracted bacterial pneumonia. The Schaibles are members of the First-Century Gospel Church, a faith healing group located in northeast Philadelphia that believes illness is a test from Satan and getting medical care is idolatry that upsets a jealous God. The Church has a school; Herbert taught seventh and eighth grades, and Catherine was the daughter of the principal. Both believed that prayer was all they needed to heal their children.

After Kent died, the jury convicted the Schaibles of manslaughter and child endangerment. Common Pleas Court Judge Carolyn Engle Temin sentenced them to ten years of probation and ordered them to get regular medical check-ups for their other seven children.

Temin was clear about what she wanted. "You are to consult a medical practitioner whenever a child exhibits signs of being sick," she said. "And you are to follow the medical practitioner's advice to the letter." Herbert's response was a warning of what was to come. "With God's help, this will never happen again," he said.

During the Schaibles' sentencing hearing following the death of Kent, Catherine's attorney, Mythri Jayaraman, expressed doubt that the couple would follow the orders of the court: "I have some concerns personally about their ability within their faith or their willingness to proactively take their children to get medical attention." Jayaraman asked the court to assign someone from the health department to monitor the children. Only healthcare workers, she argued, understood what routine medical care meant. But the court's hands were tied. Because Pennsylvania had a religious exemption to medical neglect, the Schaible children couldn't be monitored by a state health agency; only state probation officers were permitted to watch them. And they didn't know what to look for.

Between 2011 and 2013, following the death of Kent, Herbert Schaible reported to his probation officer four times. While probation officers were monitoring Herbert, Brandon never received the routine medical care Temin had ordered; he was examined by a doctor ten days after he was born and never again.

At the preliminary hearing following Brandon's death, Common Pleas Court Judge Benjamin Lerner said that by failing to seek medical care, the Schaibles had "knowingly, intentionally, callously, and hypocritically" violated their probation. The Schaibles didn't see it that way. They *had* gotten help. They'd asked the assistant pastor at their church to come to the house and pray. God was their doctor. And God had chosen to take their son. When questioned by a homicide detective, Herbert Schaible, in direct contradiction to the probation order following the death of his first child, said, "Of course we didn't take [Brandon] to a doctor."

On May 21, 2013, the coroner found that Brandon Schaible—like his brother before him—had died from bacterial pneumonia. His death was ruled a homicide. The next day, Herbert and Catherine Schaible were charged with third-degree murder, involuntary manslaughter, conspiracy, and endangerment. "I am sorry for your loss: deeply sorry," Judge Lerner told the couple. "But in all honesty, I am more sorry for the fact that this innocent little child will not be able to grow up to be what he wanted to be."

On November 14, 2013, Herbert and Catherine Schaible pled no contest to third-degree murder; on February 19, 2014, both were sentenced to 3½ to 7 years in prison, and their children were permanently placed into foster homes. "I don't have any pipeline to Heaven," said Judge Lerner, "but I do know that it wasn't God who decided to take [your son]. It was the two of you who took him." Herbert was contrite, promising that in the future he would follow the court's probationary rules "to a T."

Remarkably, while Brandon Schaible lay dying, the General Assembly of Pennsylvania continued to protect parents who use a religious defense to medical neglect charges. Senate bills 20 and 28 state: "If a child has not been provided needed medical or surgical care because of seriously held religious beliefs of the child's parents . . . *the child shall not be deemed to be physically or mentally abused.*" Although the Senate bills made it clear that child neglect was not to be tolerated, the bills also made it clear that religiously motivated child neglect would be.

The first person to rise up against Pennsylvania's repeated failure to protect children like Kent and Brandon Schaible was Rita Swan, who traveled from her home in Lexington, Kentucky, to Harrisburg. In June 2013, Swan met with five legislative staffers as well as the executive director of the Pennsylvania Children and Youth Administration, an organization representing directors of child welfare agencies.

Rita was certain that she could appeal to the executive director. It didn't work out that way. "[He] was impervious to every point I made," recalled Rita. "He was patronizing, telling me I was a bereaved mother who needed to expiate my guilt. He said that he and his people were the experts." When it comes to religious exemptions to child abuse and neglect, Pennsylvania laws are particularly troubling—it is one of only two states that allows a religious exemption to bicycle helmets, and one of only a handful of states that allow parents who refuse medical care to adopt children.

Today, parents in Pennsylvania can be sent to prison if they unreasonably restrain a child or if they drive a child while under the influence of alcohol or if they cause a child to be near a methamphetamine lab or if they slap or shake a baby. But if they withhold lifesaving medicines—and do it in the name of God—the odds are they'll never spend a day in jail. Parents can still claim a religious motive for this most unreligious act.

STATE LEGISLATORS aren't the only problem. Recently, the federal government also passed on an opportunity to stand up for children whose lives are in danger. It happened during discussions around President Obama's Affordable Care Act.

As of March 31, 2014, all United States citizens were required to have health insurance, either through the Affordable Care Act or otherwise. As was the case for CAPTA, Christian Scientists saw this as a threat to their way of life. So, on March 4, the Christian Science Church scheduled a "national call-in day" for the following week, urging members to support two identical bills: one in the House of Representatives (HR1814) and one in the Senate (S.862). Both would exempt anyone with "sincerely held religious beliefs against medical health care" from the mandate to buy health insurance. On March 11, the day of the call-in, the bill passed the House. The Congressional Budget Office estimated that the bill would increase the number of uninsured persons by five hundred thousand each year and cost $1.5 billion over ten years. More importantly, the federal government had once again lost an opportunity to protect children from parents who reject modern medicine in the name of their faith.

GIVEN THE CLARITY of the issue, why have Americans been reluctant to counter parents who neglect their children for religious reasons? Several possible explanations have been offered, some more demoralizing than others.

First, most Americans probably don't know that there's a problem—don't know that children are suffering and dying because their parents are choosing prayer instead of modern medicine. Although the media often tell these stories, only rarely do they rise above the noise of other tragedies. And most faith healing groups are quite insular, so their stories probably never get told.

Second, America was founded as a safe haven for religious beliefs that weren't tolerated elsewhere. For this reason, the First Amendment was designed to keep the federal government out of the business of making laws regarding religion. Unfortunately, the American public's instinctive tolerance for religion often exceeds reason—in this case, resulting in a misguided respect for a belief that violates one of the most fundamental teachings of all religions: protecting the vulnerable.

Third, and most worrisome, Americans have always been proud of their autonomy, particularly in the family realm. There's a certain libertarian streak in American jurisprudence—we don't like to be told what to do. Evidence for this can be found in the reaction by the United States government to the United Nations Convention on the Rights of the Child.

In 1989, the United Nations drafted a document specifically outlining the rights of the world's children. The Convention acknowledged that all children had the right to life, the right to be protected from abuse and exploitation, the right to be exempt from capital punishment, and the right to be protected from cruel or degrading forms of corporal punishment. More than 190 countries signed this document, including almost every member of the United Nations. Only two countries refused: Somalia and the United States. Most observers believe that the reason that the United States has refused to sign this document is that Americans don't like to be told how to raise their children. President Obama called his country's refusal to ratify the Convention "embarrassing."

EPILOGUE

"THE FRAIL WEB OF UNDERSTANDING"

"Our only hope lies in the frail web of understanding
of one person for the pain of another."

—John Dos Passos, American novelist

On the evening of March 16, 2012, Dr. Robert W. Block, president of the American Academy of Pediatrics, handed a plaque to Rita Swan—the President's Certificate for Outstanding Service. Block announced that Swan was being recognized for "personal dedication to the health, safety, and wellbeing of children." "Thanks so much for this wonderful award," said Rita. "It will always be on a wall in our home."

It wasn't the first time the Academy had bestowed its most prestigious award. Every year for decades, the president would stand in front of a national audience of pediatricians and hand it out. Usually the award was given to doctors. But Swan wasn't a doctor. She was a mother who had held her child in her arms while he died of meningitis—a treatable illness she had refused to treat. Day after day, while her son suffered high fevers and seizures before eventually slipping into a coma, Rita Swan prayed—prayed until the bacteria that were infecting his brain and spinal cord overwhelmed him—prayed even though the antibiotics that would have saved his life were only a car ride away.

During her twenty-minute acceptance speech, Swan talked mostly about her efforts to stop other parents from doing what she had done; efforts that had consumed her for more than three decades; efforts that had caused her to spend many sleepless nights knowing that medical neglect in the name of God was still happening. And that it was still being allowed to happen. Knowing that no matter how much she did, it would never be enough—that it would never bring back her son. "You never reach a point of acceptance," said Rita. "You never get past the guilt."

AN ANALOGY TO RITA SWAN's story can be found in M. Night Shyamalan's 2004 movie *The Village*—the story of an insular community united by fear. Brought together by the murder of loved ones, several Philadelphians decide to create a nineteenth-century farming community in rural Pennsylvania. Solace, they believe, could be found by retreating into the past. To isolate the community from a world they fear, the elders create mythical monsters that are supposedly hiding in the woods: referred to as "The Things Of Which We Do Not Speak." The monsters won't bother the villagers as long as the villagers don't enter the woods. As a consequence, no one enters or leaves the village. Then something happens that the elders hadn't anticipated: a young man is stabbed. When an infection develops, the only way to save him is with antibiotics. Unfortunately, the community has been created to mimic the late 1800s, a time before antibiotics. Knowing the monsters are a hoax, the elders allow one of the residents, a young woman, to travel through the woods and get the antibiotics they need. They pick her because she's blind—hoping that when she returns, she won't have realized the wealth of lifesaving technologies on the other side.

Religions that ask their followers to act against love, compassion, and reason use a similar tactic. Rita Swan was afraid to oppose her church and see a doctor because her church believed that doctors want "to dethrone God" and are therefore evil. If she had sought out modern medicine, she would have been forced to confront that evil and, worse, the anger of God. But Rita Swan wasn't blind. When she crossed the woods and entered the Wayne State University Medical Library—and understood how she could have treated her son's illness—there was no going back, even if it meant ostracism from a community she had known all her life, even if it meant challenging her notion of God. Swan's break with her church came when she realized that *no* God would ask a parent to let a child die in His name.

"I believe that the Sabbath was made for man and not man for the Sabbath," said Swan. "That's what Jesus says. So I think religion has to work. It has to bless people. And if it doesn't, if it causes pain, if it justifies cruelty, then it's something I don't want any part of. I think we have to be explicit in rejecting things that are cruel and unjust whether they're religious or not. Religion has to serve the good of humanity."

Not the other way around.

"IF MAN IS CREATED in the likeness of God," writes Erich Fromm in *Escape From Freedom*, "he is the bearer of infinite qualities." Fromm argues that organized religions act most egregiously, most destructively, and most inhumanely when they ignore the beauty of Genesis 1:27: *So God created man in His own image, in the image of God He created him; male and female He created them.* In other words, people should see in themselves the rich and infinite powers of love and reason that God has bestowed upon them. This is exactly what Rita Swan did when she ventured through the woods of her fears and walked into a medical library. And what she continues to do by fighting for the rights of children every day. In the end, Rita Swan didn't need to be motivated by fear of God's reprisal or God's reward for her virtue; she was motivated to do the right thing because it was the right thing to do. It was in that way that she has best served God.

NOTES

Introduction: At the Crossroads

ix   **The death of Brandon Schaible:** M. Newall, "Couple Probed in Death of 2d Child," *Philadelphia Inquirer*, April 20, 2013; M. Newall, "Second Ill Child of Devout Parents Dies," *Philadelphia Inquirer*, April 23, 2013; M. Newall, "Schaibles' Oversight Was Issue in 2011," *Philadelphia Inquirer*, April 24, 2013; M. Newall, "Pastor: 'Spiritual Lack' Killed Two Boys," *Philadelphia Inquirer*, April 28, 2013; M. Newall, "Death of Faith-Healing Couple's Baby Is Ruled Homicide," *Philadelphia Inquirer*, May 22, 2013; S. Leach, "M. E.: Death of Faith-Healing Couple's Baby Is Murder," *Philadelphia Daily News*, May 22, 2013; M. Dribben, "Schaible Couple Denied Release," *Philadelphia Inquirer*, May 25, 2013; "Pennsylvania Religious Objectors Lose a Second Baby," *Children's Healthcare Is a Legal Duty* newsletter, Number 1, 2013.

ix   **Faith healing sects in the United States:** S. M. Asser and R. Swan, "Child Fatalities from Religion-Motivated Medical Neglect," *Pediatrics* 101 (1998): 625–629.

x   **Jehovah's Witness who regretted transfusion:** Katie Cantore, personal communication, May 16, 2013.

x   **Terrance Cottrell Jr.:** Peters, *When Prayer Fails*, 203–212; D. Reynolds, "Boy Dies as Churchgoers Try To Remove 'Evil Spirits' of Autism," *Inclusion Daily Express*, August 27, 2003; M. Davey, "Exorcism Death Sparks Debate," *The Charlotte Observer*, August 29, 2003; D. Reynolds, "Pastor Pleads Not Guilty To Abusing Junior Cottrell," *Inclusion Daily Express*, September 18, 2003; D. Reynolds, "Hemphill Sentenced Over Boy's 'Exorcism' Death," *Inclusion Daily Express*, August 20, 2004; R. Swan, "Minister Sentenced in Fatal Exorcism," *Children's Healthcare Is a Legal Duty* newsletter, Number 3, 2004.

x   **Baltimore exorcism conference:** L. Goodstein, "For Catholics, Interest in Exorcism Is Revived," *New York Times*, November 12, 2010.

xi   **Spitting blood:** "Metzitzah B'Peh: Oral Law?" *Ideals*, Institute for Jewish Idea and Ideals, www.jewishideas.org/print/498.

xi   **Herpes virus cases following circumcision:** "Metzitzah B'Peh: Oral Law?" *Ideals*, Institute for Jewish Idea and Ideals, www.jewishideas.org/print/498; L. Robbins, "Baby's Death Removes Debate Over a Circumcision Ritual," *New York Times*, March 7, 2012; "New York, Orthodox Jews Clash Over Circumcision," *National Public Radio*, December 3, 2012, http://npr.org /news/U.S./166399479; S. D. James, "Herpes Strikes Infants After Ritual Circumcision," *ABC News*, April 5, 2013, http://abcnews.go.com/m /story?id=18890284.

xi   **Measles outbreak in Texas:** J. Aleccia, "Measles Outbreak Tied to Texas Megachurch Sickens 21," *NBC News*, August 27, 2013; T. Culp-Ressler, "Measles Outbreak Linked to Texas Megachurch Whose Pastor Has Spread Myths About Vaccines," *ThinkProgress*, August 27, 2013, http://think progress.org/health/2013/08/27/2532651/measles-outbreak-texas-mega church; J. Stengle, "Measles Cases Put Texas Megachurch Under Scrutiny," *Associated Press*, August 31, 2013; "Texas Megachurch at Center of Measles Outbreak," *National Public Radio*, September 1, 2013.

xii **Abortion in a Catholic hospital:** B. B. Hagerty, "Nun Excommunicated for Allowing Abortion," *National Public Radio*, May 19, 2010, www.npr.org /templates/story/story.php?storyid=126985072; "Nun Excommunicated: Loses Hospital Post Over Decision on Abortion," Catholic News Service, May 18, 2010, www.catholicnews.com/data/stories/cns/1002085 .htm; "Statements from the Diocese of Phoenix," *Arizona Republic*, May 15, 2010, www.azcentral.com/community/phoenix/articles/2010/05/14 /20100514stjoseph0515bishop.html.

xii **Catholic hospitals in the United States:** B. Garrison, "Playing Catholic Politics with U.S. Healthcare," *The Guardian*, December 31, 2010.

Chapter 1: "The Very Worst Thing"

Unless otherwise noted, all of Rita Swan's quotes were obtained from an interview with the author on May 22, 2013.

2   **Mary Baker Eddy's youth:** Nickell, *Looking for a Miracle*, 154; Fraser, *God's Perfect Child*, 26.

2   **Eddy's mother and the Divine Spirit:** Fraser, *God's Perfect Child*, 29.

2   **Eddy's psychosomatic illnesses:** Ibid., 34–35.

2   **Biographer regarding Eddy's psychosomatic illnesses:** Ibid., 35.

2   **Eddy regarding frogs and sawdust:** Cather and Milmine, *Life of Mary Baker Eddy*, 34.

2–3   **Eddy's use of heteropathic healers and her first encounter with Phineas Parkhurst Quimby:** Schoefplin, *Christian Science on Trial*, 22–24.

3   **Quimby's philosophy:** Ibid., 24; Porterfield, *Healing in the History of Christianity*, 178–179; Rose, *Faith Healing*, 62–64; Fraser, *God's Perfect Child*, 42–51.

3   **Eddy's epiphany:** Schoefplin, *Christian Science on Trial*, 23.

3   **Eddy as psychic medium:** Cather and Milmine, *Life of Mary Baker Eddy*, 30.

4   **Eddy's philosophy:** Nickell, *Looking for a Miracle*, 155; Porterfield, *Healing in the History of Christianity*, 178; Jenny, *Child Abuse and Neglect*, 599; Eddy, *Science and Health with Key to the Scriptures*.

4   **Eddy's philosophy contrasted to Quimby's:** Porterfield, *Healing in the History of Christianity*, 179; Fraser, *God's Perfect Child*, 47–51.

4   **Christian Science vs. Christianity:** Ibid., 68–69; Kramer, *Religion that Kills*, 68–69.

4   **Christian Science vs. science:** R. Swan, *Children's Healthcare Is a Legal Duty* newsletter, Number 3, 2004.

4   **Success of Christian Science:** Fraser, *God's Perfect Child*, 15–16.

5   **Ben Franklin regarding faith healing:** Ibid., 48.

5   **Anatomist regarding state of medicine:** Ibid., 48.

5   **Eddy rejects the germ theory:** R. Swan, "Fragile and Belligerent Magic: Religious Beliefs Against Medical Care," *Kentucky Hospitals*, Winter 1989.

9   **Doug Swan regarding Rita's suspension from Sunday school:** *The Phil Donohue Show*, May 15, 1988.

10–18   **Matthew Swan story:** R. Swan, *The Last Strawberry*.

18   **Christian Science official states the Swans were free to see a doctor:** B. Bell, "Their Baby's Death Provokes Doug and Rita Swan to a Holy War on Christian Science," *People*, March 31, 1980.

Chapter 2: A Fragile Magic

19   **Doug Swan regarding taking Matthew to a doctor:** *PBS Late Night* with Dennis Wholley, May 1982.

19 **Rita Swan regarding practitioners:** *Kelly and Company, WXYZ*, Detroit, *ABC TV*, May 1982.

19 **Doug Swan regarding breaking commandments:** *PBS Late Night* with Dennis Wholley, May 1982; *Court TV* with Catherine Crier, July 31, 2000.

20 **Christian Science is a healthcare system:** *Crossroads* with Charles Kurault and Bill Moyers, *CBS Network*, June 27, 1984.

20 **Norman Fost regarding holding Christian Science practitioner accountable:** *Nightline* with Ted Koppel, *ABC TV*, June 17, 1988.

20 **Rita Swan regarding moral responsibility:** *Crossroads* with Charles Kurault and Bill Moyers, *CBS Network*, June 27, 1984; *Nightline* with Ted Koppel, *ABC TV*, June 17, 1988.

20 **Doug Swan regarding guilt:** *The Phil Donohue Show*, May 17, 1988.

21 **Rita Swan regarding vulnerability:** *Kelly and Company, WXYZ*, Detroit, *ABC TV*, May 1982.

21 **Doug Swan regarding television:** *Crossroads* with Charles Kurault and Bill Moyers, *CBS Network*, June 27, 1984.

21 **Doug Swan regarding ignorance as an advantage:** *People Are Talking* with Nancy Merrill, *WBZ*, Boston, *NBC TV*, May 23, 1984.

21 **Rita Swan regarding PhD and ignorance:** Ibid.

21 **Rita Swan regarding isolation:** *Kelly and Company, WXYZ*, Detroit, *ABC TV*, May 1982.

21 **Hobart Freeman and the Faith Assembly Church:** *WJW*, Cleveland, *When Faith Is Fatal*, five-part series airing the week of November 13, 1987, *FOX TV*; R. Swan, *Children's Healthcare Is a Legal Duty* newsletter, Summer 1986.

22 **Natali Joy Mudd:** Peters, *When Prayer Fails*, 16; J. Quinn and B. Zlatos, "52 Deaths Tied to Sect," *Fort Wayne (IN) News-Sentinel*, May 2, 1983.

22 **Walter White and the Followers of Christ Church:** *ABC's 20/20*, May 6, 1988; M. Larabee and P. D. Sleeth, "Followers Children Needed Medical Care, Experts Say," *The (Cleveland, OH) Plain Dealer*, June 28, 1998.

22 **Neil Beagley:** R. Swan, "Followers' of Christ Parents Sentenced to Prison in Son's Death," *Children's Healthcare Is a Legal Duty* newsletter, Number 1, 2010.

23 **Jim Jones and the People's Temple:** Scheeres, *A Thousand Lives*.

25 **David Koresh and the Branch Davidians:** Linedecker, *Massacre at Waco*; Tabor and Gallagher, *Why Waco*.

26 **Marshall Applewhite and Heaven's Gate:** Perkins and Jackson, *Cosmic Suicide*.

29   **Eddy likens herself to Jesus:** Kramer, *Religion that Kills*, 68–69.

29   **Robert Jay Lifton and cults:** Lifton, *Thought Reform*, 419–437.

32   **Faith healing sects in the United States:** S. M. Asser and R. Swan, "Child Fatalities from Religion-Motivated Medical Neglect," *Pediatrics* 101 (1998): 625–629.

Chapter 3: A Vengeful God

35   **Rita Swan regarding concept of God:** R. Swan, *The Last Strawberry*.

35   **Stanley Milgram regarding obedience in Nazi Germany:** Milgram, *Obedience to Authority*, 1.

36   **Milgram experiment:** Ibid.

39–40   **Hannah Arendt regarding Eichmann:** Arendt, *Eichmann in Jerusalem*.

Chapter 4: The Faith Healer Next Door

43   **Story of Larry and Lucky Parker:** Parker, *We Let Our Son Die*.

54   **Dependent Personality Disorder:** Dobbert, *Understanding Personality Disorders*; American Psychiatric Association, *DSM-5*.

55   **Narcissistic Personality Disorder:** Ibid.

57   **Oral Roberts' claims of resurrections:** Randi, *Faith Healers*, 256.

58   **Parker believes that faith healers are influenced by the devil:** Parker, *No Spin Faith*, 26.

58   **Parker states that his mission is to prevent others from doing what he did:** Parker, *No Spin Faith*, 20.

58   **Parker criticizes Kenneth Copeland:** Parker, *No Spin Faith*, 54.

Chapter 5: The Literal and the Damned

59   **Larry Parker regarding God:** Parker, *We Let Our Son Die*.

61–63   **The exorcism and death of Terrance Cottrell Jr.:** Peters, *When Prayer Fails*, 203–212; D. Reynolds, "Boy Dies as Churchgoers Try To Remove 'Evil Spirits' of Autism," *Inclusion Daily Express*, August 27, 2003; M. Davey, "Exorcism Death Sparks Debate," *The Charlotte Observer*, August 29, 2003; D. Reynolds, "Pastor Pleads Not Guilty To Abusing Junior Cottrell," *Inclusion Daily Express*, September 18, 2003; D. Reynolds, "Hemphill Sentenced Over Boy's 'Exorcism' Death," *Inclusion Daily Express*, August 20, 2004; R. Swan, "Minister Sentenced in Fatal Exorcism," *Children's Healthcare Is a Legal Duty* newsletter, Number 3, 2004.

63 ***The Possession:*** T. Tugend, "In Hollywood's 'The Possession,' the Dybbuk Is Back," *Jewish Telegraphic Agency*, August 29, 2012.

64 ***The Exorcist:*** A. Breznican, "The Exorcist: 10 Creepy Details from the Scariest Movie Ever Made," *Entertainment Weekly*, October 31, 2012.

64 **Pope Paul VI and Satan:** Randi, *Faith Healers*, 79.

64 **Gallop and Pew polls:** C. Fraser, "Ancient and Modern Exorcism, Alias Laying On of Hands, Denounced," *Children's Healthcare is a Legal Duty* newsletter, Number 2, 2009; C. M. Blow, "Bobby Jindal, the Exorcist," *New York Times*, February 28, 2009.

64 **Gwinnett County case:** C. Fraser, "Ancient and Modern Exorcism, Alias Laying On of Hands, Denounced," *Children's Healthcare is a Legal Duty* newsletter, Number 2, 2009.

64 **Popularity of exorcism:** Cuneo, *American Exorcism*.

64–65 **Baltimore exorcism conference:** L. Goodstein, "For Catholics, Interest in Exorcism Is Revived," *New York Times*, November 12, 2010.

65 **Exorcism of Anneliese Michel:** Randi, *Faith Healers*, 80; "Exorcism," *The Skeptic's Dictionary*, Skeptic.com.

66 **Exorcism deaths:** "Exorcism," *The Skeptic's Dictionary*, Skeptic.com.

66 **Exorcism death in Maryland:** F. Karimi and J. Sutton, "Police: Maryland Mom Kills 2 of Her Children During Attempted Exorcism," *CNN*, January 9, 2014.

66 **Ray Hemphill's sentence:** Hamilton, *God vs. Gavel*, 40.

66 **Description of circumcision:** S. Otterman, "Denouncing City's Move to Regulate Circumcision," *New York Times*, September 12, 2012.

67 **Babylonian Talmud regarding circumcision:** B. Gesundheit, G. Srisaru-Soen, D. Greenberg, et al., "Neonatal Genital Herpes Simplex Virus Type 1 Infection After Jewish Ritual Circumcision: Modern Medicine and Religious Tradition," *Pediatrics* 114 (2004): e259-e263.

67 ***Yoreh Deah* regarding spitting blood:** "Metzitzah B'Peh: Oral Law?" *Ideals*, Institute for Jewish Idea and Ideals, www.jewishideas.org/print/498.

68 ***Metzitzah* causes tuberculosis and syphilis:** E. L. Lewis, "Tuberculosis of the Penis: A Report of 5 New Cases, and a Complete Review of the Literature," *Journal of Urology* 56 (1946): 737–45; B. L. Leas, C. A. Umscheid, "Neonatal Herpes Simplex Virus Type 1 Infection and Jewish Ritual Circumcision with Oral Suction: A Systematic Review," *Journal*

of the Pediatric Infectious Diseases Society (2014): 1–6, DOI: 10.1093/jpids /piu075.

68 **Rabbi Moses Schreiber regarding use of sterile instruments:**
B. Gesundheit, G. Srisaru-Soen, D. Greenberg, et al., "Neonatal Genital
Herpes Simplex Virus Type 1 Infection After Jewish Ritual Circumcision:
Modern Medicine and Religious Tradition," *Pediatrics* 114 (2004): e259-e263.

69 **Herpes infections linked to *mohel*:** L. Robbins, "Baby's Death Removes
Debate Over a Circumcision Ritual," *New York Times*, March 7, 2012;
Centers for Disease Control and Prevention, "Neonatal Herpes Simplex
Virus Infection Following Jewish Ritual Circumcisions that Included Direct
Orogenital Suction—New York City, 2000–2011," *Morbidity and Mortality
Weekly Report* 61 (2012): 405–409.

69 **CDC statement regarding sterile technique:** Centers for Disease Control
and Prevention, "Neonatal Herpes Simplex Virus Infection Following Jewish
Ritual Circumcisions that Included Direct Orogenital Suction—New York
City, 2000–2011," *Morbidity and Mortality Weekly Report* 61 (2012):
405–409.

69 **New York City mayor Michael Bloomberg regarding *metzitzah*:**
L. Robbins, "Baby's Death Removes Debate Over a Circumcision Ritual,"
New York Times, March 7, 2012.

69 **Number of infants in New York City subjected to *metzitzah*:** S. Otterman,
"Denouncing City's Move to Regulate Circumcision," *New York Times*,
September 12, 2012.

69–70 **New York City law regulating *metzitzah*:** C. Nordqvist, "Infection Risk
Prompts New York City to Approve Ritual Circumcision Laws," *Medical
News Today*, September 16, 2012.

70 **Romi Cohn objects to regulation:** "New York, Orthodox Jews
Clash Over Circumcision," *National Public Radio*, December 3, 2012,
http://npr.org/news/U.S./166399479.

70 **Rabbi David Niederman regarding change:** L. Robbins, "Baby's Death
Removes Debate Over a Circumcision Ritual," *New York Times*, March 7, 2012.

70 **Isaac Mortob regarding males being fully Jewish:** S. Otterman,
"Denouncing City's Move to Regulate Circumcision," *New York Times*,
September 12, 2012.

70 **Ultra-Orthodox rabbis regarding health department's plans:** J. Allen,
"New Rule Angers Some in Orthodox Community," *Reuters*, September 13,
2012.

70   **Rabbis regarding violation of constitutional rights:** "Rabbis Challenge NYC Over Controversial Circumcision," *CBS/Associated Press*, October 12, 2012, www.cbsnews.com/8301–204_162–57531340/rabbis-challenge-nyc-over -controversial-circumcision.

70   **Dr. William Schaffner regarding modern science:** S. D. James, "Baby Dies of Herpes in Ritual Circumcision by Orthodox Jews," *ABC News*, March 12, 2012, http://abcnews.go.com/Health/baby-dies-herpes-virus -ritual-circumcision-nyc-orthodox/story?id=15888618.

70   **Dr. Jay Varma regarding *metzitzah*:** S. Otterman, "Denouncing City's Move to Regulate Circumcision," *New York Times*, September 12, 2012.

71   **Rabbi Moshe Tendler regarding *metzitzah*:** P. Kim, "Circumcision Ritual Under Fire in New York Due to Risk of Herpes Infection," *CNN*, July 7, 2012, http://religion.blogs.cnn.com/2012/07/07/circumcision-under-fire -in-new-york-due-to-risk-of-herpes-infection.

71   **Rabbi Gerald Skolnik regarding Jewish tradition:** S. Otterman, "Denouncing City's Move to Regulate Circumcision," *New York Times*, September 12, 2012.

71   **Chief Rabbinate of Israel regarding *metzitzah*:** B. Gesundheit, G. Srisaru-Soen, D. Greenberg, et al., "Neonatal Genital Herpes Simplex Virus Type 1 Infection After Jewish Ritual Circumcision: Modern Medicine and Religious Tradition," *Pediatrics* 114 (2004): e259-e263.

71–72   ***Metzitzah* is against Jewish law:** I. Youngster, B. Z. Katz, "Tradition . . . Tradition . . . " *Journal of the Pediatric Infectious Diseases Society* (2014): 1–2, DOI:10.1093/jpids/piu082.

72   **Judge rules against rabbis; three more herpes cases:** S. D. James, "Herpes Strikes Infants After Ritual Circumcision," *ABC News*, April 5, 2013, http: //abcnews.go.com/m/story?id=18890284; J. A. Schillinger and S. Blank, "2014 Alert #2," New York City Department of Health and Mental Hygiene, January 28, 2014.

72   **Herpes virus infections in New Jersey:** D. N. Cohen, "Two Babies Sickened by Circumcision Rite," Forward.com, March 23, 2012, http://forward.com /articles/153089/two-babies-sickened-by-circumcision-right/?p=all.

Chapter 6: Dialogue of the Deaf

75   **"Dialogue of the deaf":** G. O'Brien, *The Church and Abortion*, 147.

77   **Judith Woods regarding when life begins:** S. Ditum, "After Savita Halappanavar's Death, the Brutal Irony of 'Pro-Life' Is Exposed," *The Guardian*, November 19, 2012.

77   **Tertullian regarding abortion:** Scarnecchia, *Bioethics, Law, and Human Rights*, 276.

77   **Pope John Paul II and Archbishop Chaput regarding abortion:** G. O'Brien, *The Church and Abortion*, 6, 10.

77   **Vatican Council II regarding abortion:** Scarnecchia, *Bioethics, Law, and Human Rights*, 280.

78   **Brian Scarnecchia regarding abortion:** Ibid., 274–275.

78   **Severity of unnamed mother's illness:** B. B. Hagerty, "Nun Excommunicated for Allowing Abortion," *National Public Radio*, May 19, 2010, www.npr.org/templates/story/story.php?storyid=126985072.

79   **Sister Margaret McBride's background:** "Sister Margaret McBride: VP of Organizational Outreach," *Catholic Healthcare West*, 2013, www.st josephs-phx.org/Who_We_Are/208291.

79   **Bishop Thomas Olmsted regarding abortion as an evil:** "Nun Excommunicated, Loses Hospital Post Over Decision on Abortion," *Catholic News Service*, May 18, 2010, www.catholicnews.com/data /stories/cns/1002085.htm.

79   **Statement from Linda Hunt:** A. L. Myers, "Ariz. Hospital Loses Catholic Status Over Surgery," *Seattle Times*, December 21, 2010.

80   **Statement from Catholic Healthcare West:** "Nun Excommunicated, Loses Hospital Post Over Decision on Abortion," *Catholic News Service*, May 18, 2010, www.catholicnews.com/data/stories/cns/1002085.htm.

80   **Statement by Bishop Olmsted regarding Pope John Paul II's decree:** "Statements from the Diocese of Phoenix," *Arizona Republic*, May 15, 2010, www.azcentral.com/community/phoenix/articles/2010/05/14 /20100514stjoseph0515bishop.html.

81   **Gianna Beretta Molla:** Scarnecchia, *Bioethics, Law, and Human Life Issues*, 273–274.

82   **Savita Halappanavar background:** G. Chamberlain, "'Change Your Abortion Laws to Save Lives,' Grieving Father Tells Irish PM," *The Guardian*, November 17, 2012.

82   **Father regarding Savita Halappanavar's pregnancy:** Ibid.

82   **Praveen Halappanavar regarding Savita's pregnancy:** S. Pollak, "Ireland's Historic Abortion Shift and the Tragedy that Shadowed It," *World Time*,

December 19, 2012, world.time.com/2012/12/19/Ireland-historic-abortion -shift-and-the-tragedy-that-shadowed-it/print.

82–83 Praveen Halappanavar regarding Savita's early hospital course:
H. McDonald and B. Quinn, "Ireland's Abortion Policy Under Scrutiny After Woman's Death," *The Guardian*, November 14, 2012; "Indian Woman's Death in Ireland Sparks Debate Over Abortion," *Associated Press*, November 15, 2012.

83–84 Praveen Halappanavar regarding Savita's downhill course: Ibid.

84 Praveen Halappanavar regarding Savita's death: Ibid.

84 Savita Halappanavar's autopsy: K. Holland, "HIQA Names Members of Investigation Team," *Irish Times*, December 20, 2012.

84 Savita Halappanavar's father regarding Savita: G. Chamberlain, "Change Your Abortion Laws to Save Lives, Grieving Father Tells Irish PM," *The Guardian*, November 17, 2012.

84 Praveen Halappanavar regarding Savita: S. Pollak, "Ireland's Historic Abortion Shift and the Tragedy that Shadowed It," *World Time*, December 19, 2012, world.time.com/2012/12/19/Ireland-historic-abortion-shift-and-the-tragedy-that-shadowed-it/print.

84 Praveen Halappanavar regarding family's reaction to Savita's death: Ibid.

84 Savita Halappanavar's mother reacts to death: "Savita Halappanavar's Parents Slam Irish Abortion Laws," *Associated Press*, November 15, 2012.

84–85 *Times of India* editorial: H. McDonald, "Savita Halappanavar 'Would Still Be Alive if She Had Been Treated in India,'" *The Guardian*, November 16, 2012.

85 Marches in Ireland: G. Horgan, "Savita Halappanavar's Death Has Transformed Irish Abortion Debate," *The Guardian*, November 16, 2012; H. McDonald, "Thousands March in Dublin Over Abortion Rights," *The Guardian*, November 17, 2012.

85 Response from Catholic Bishops of Ireland: "Treatment That Risks Fetus Can Be 'Ethically Permissible'—Catholic Bishops," www.rte.ie/ news/2012/1119/x-case-legislation-abortion.html.

85 Irish women travel to England for abortions: "Savita Halappanavar's Parents Slam Irish Abortion Laws," *Associated Press*, November 15, 2012.

85 Edna Kenny and changing Ireland's abortion laws: J. Lindsay, "Cardinal Skipping BC Ceremony Over Abortion Issue," *Associated Press*, May 10, 2013.

85 **Protection of Life During Pregnancy Act:** "Controversial Irish Abortion Law Comes Into Effect," *RT News*, http://rt.com/news/ireland-abortion -law-force-060.

86 **Brazilian case of rape and incest:** F. X. Rocca, "Vatican Official Defends Child's Abortion," *Washington Post*, March 21, 2009.

86 **Archbishop Cardoso Sobrinho regarding laws of man versus laws of God:** "Brazil Church Excommunicates Mom, Doctors After Raped 9-Year-Old Has Abortion," www.foxnews.com/story/0,2933,505183,00 .html.

86 **Archbishop Sobrinho regarding stepfather:** J. Smits, "Mgr. Cardoso, Archbishop of Recife: Exclusive Interview in 'Présent,'" *Riposte Catholique*, May 30, 2009.

86–87 **Archbishop Salvatore Fisichella's comments:** J. Brown, "Brazil's Bishops Beleaguered But Blessed," March 23, 2009, www.renewamerica.com /columns/brown/090323; F. X. Rocca, "Vatican Official Defends Child's Abortion," *Washington Post*, March 21, 2009; C. Glatz, "Church Credibility Harmed by 'Hasty' Excommunication," *National Catholic Reporter*, March 16, 2009.

87 **George O'Brien regarding rape and incest:** G. O'Brien, *Church and Abortion*, 85.

88–89 **Kyle Smith regarding *Philomena*:** K. Smith, "'*Philomena*' Another Hateful and Boring Attack on Catholics," *New York Post*, November 21, 2013.

89 **Vatican official supports Sobrinho:** J. Israely, "A Sequel to the Case of the Pregnant 9-Year Old," *Time*, July 18, 2009.

Chapter 7: Do Unto Others

All retrospective quotes from Dr. Robert Ross were obtained from an interview on May 29, 2013.

91–92 **Michael Heilman:** Peters, *When Prayer Fails*, 3–8.

92 **Measles enters Philadelphia:** R. Palley, "Disease Is Easily Prevented With Free Shot But 35,000 Pre-Schoolers Aren't Protected," *Philadelphia Daily News*, February 12, 1991; S. Fitzgerald, "Measles a Sign of System's Failure: Government, Doctors and Even Parents Have Failed to Make Childhood Shots a Priority, A Report Says," *Philadelphia Inquirer*, March 10, 1991.

92 **Measles epidemic:** M. Schogol, "No Measley Problem," *Philadelphia Inquirer*, May 21, 1990.

92–93 **Measles disease and epidemiology:** *Epidemiology and Prevention of Vaccine-Preventable Diseases*, W. Atkinson, L. Furphy, J. Gantt, M. Mayfield, G. Rhyne (eds.), Centers for Disease Control and Prevention, 3rd Edition, January, 1996.

93 **Lack of measles immunizations:** M. Schogol, "Measles Deaths," *Philadelphia Inquirer*, June 2, 1990.

93 **CDC changes vaccine recommendation:** "State Urges Second Measles Shot for Children," *Philadelphia Inquirer*, June 12, 1990.

93 **Measles epidemic in Philadelphia, 1990:** S. Fitzgerald, "Epidemic Looms, So. Phila. Plans to Accelerate Measles Vaccination," *Philadelphia Inquirer*, November 29, 1990; L. Copeland, "Shots Urged in Warning on Measles," *Philadelphia Inquirer*, December 7, 1990; S. Fitzgerald, "N. Phila. Baby Death Linked to Measles," *Philadelphia Inquirer*, January 16, 1991.

94 **Philadelphia child dies of measles pneumonia:** S. Fitzgerald, "N. Phila. Baby Death Linked to Measles," *Philadelphia Inquirer*, January 16, 1991.

94 **Second Philadelphia child dies of measles:** R. Palley, "Disease Is Easily Prevented with Free Shot But 35,000 Pre-Schoolers Aren't Protected," *Philadelphia Daily News*, February 12, 1991.

94 **Philadelphia health officials recommend measles vaccine at six months of age:** S. Fitzgerald, "Epidemic Looms, So. Phila. Plans to Accelerate Measles Vaccination, *Philadelphia Inquirer*, November 29, 1990.

94–95 **Caryn Still's death:** P. Landry, "Measles Kills 2 Church School Pupils," *Philadelphia Inquirer*, February 11, 1991.

95 **Pastors refuse interviews:** J. P. Blake, "Congregants Believe God Cures All Ills," *Philadelphia Daily News*, February 12, 1991.

95 **Gordon Korn's philosophy:** Ibid.

95 **Doctrine of Philadelphia's Faith Tabernacle Congregation:** Ibid.; M. E. Ruane, "Church Believes in Healing Through Faith," *Philadelphia Inquirer*, February 12, 1991; J. P. Blake, "'Cult' Image Disturbing, Media Seen As Fueling Public Misunderstanding," *Philadelphia Daily News*, February 22, 1991.

95 **Other deaths in Faith Tabernacle Congregation:** J. P. Blake, "Congregants Believe God Cures All Ills," *Philadelphia Daily News*, February 12, 1991; M. Costantinou, "City Finds No New Measles, Health Officials To Remain Alert," *Philadelphia Daily News*, February 13, 1991.

96   **Philadelphia health commissioner Dr. Robert Sharrar closes school:**
     J. McGuire, L. Jackson, "2 Dead As Measles Shuts Church School,"
     Philadelphia Daily News, February 11, 1991.

96   **Monica Johnson's death:** Ibid.; P. Landry, "Measles Kills 2 Church School
     Pupils," *Philadelphia Inquirer*, February 11, 1991; M. Costantinou, "Victim's
     Dad: God Chose to Make Monica Sick," *Philadelphia Daily News*, February
     12, 1991.

97   **Philadelphia health commissioner Robert Ross and public health nurse
     Hazel Gilstrop call homes:** M. Costantinou, "Victim's Dad: God Chose to
     Make Monica Sick," *Philadelphia Daily News*, February 12, 1991; H.
     Goldman, M. E. Ruane, and S. Fitzgerald, "City Fears 90 Measles Cases at
     Church School," *Philadelphia Inquirer*, February 12, 1991.

97–98 **Ross visits homes:** H. Goldman, S. Fitzgerald, "Checking Measles Cases
     With a Quick Glance," *Philadelphia Inquirer*, February 13, 1991.

98   **Linette Milnes' death:** S. Fitzgerald, D. Rubin, "Cheltenham Girl, 14, Is
     Third Measles Victim," *Philadelphia Inquirer*, February 15, 1991.

98   **Philadelphia district attorney Ron Castille:** S. Fitzgerald, T. J. Gibbons Jr.,
     and K. Holmes, "2 Girls Die," *Philadelphia Inquirer*, February 16, 1991.

99   **Ross compels medical examinations:** J. P. Blake and K. Caparella,
     "2 More Measles Deaths," *Philadelphia Daily News*, February 16, 1991.

99   **Philadelphia mayor Wilson Goode threatens to request a court order
     requiring measles vaccinations:** Ibid.

100 **Dr. Mark Joffe heads the St. Christopher's team:** D. Rubin, "Measles
     Epidemic Spurs a Rush of Doctor Visits," *Philadelphia Inquirer*, February 17,
     1991.

100 **Dr. Maura Cooper heads The Children's Hospital of Philadelphia team:**
     Ibid.

100–101 **Deaths of Nancy Evans and Tina Louise Johnson:** R. Palley, K. Heine,
     "Measles Eyed in 2 More Kids' Deaths," *Philadelphia Daily News*, February
     15, 1991.

101 **CDC investigates outbreak:** S. Fitzgerald, T. J. Gibbons Jr., and
     K. Holmes, "2 Girls Die," *Philadelphia Inquirer*, February 16, 1991.

101 **Reverend Charles Reinert maintains his faith:** M. Owen, "Its Children
     Stricken with Measles, Church Puts Faith in God's Healing," *Philadelphia
     Inquirer*, February 18, 1991.

101 **Two children hospitalized by court order:** I. M. Diaz and D. Santiago,
     "Phila. Compels Hospitalization in Measles Case," *Philadelphia Inquirer*,

February 18, 1991; E. Moran, L. Jackson, and K. Heine, "Court Orders Care, City Orders Measles Victim to Hospital," *Philadelphia Daily News*, February 18, 1991; S. Fitzgerald, "City Sees Measles Subsiding But 23 From Churches Still Ill," *Philadelphia Inquirer*, February 19, 1991.

103 **Burden of measles on local hospitals:** K. Caparella, "Deaths Spur Many to Get Measles Shot," *Philadelphia Daily News*, February 19, 1991.

103 **Ross predicts more deaths:** Ibid.

104 **Two more children hospitalized by court order:** K. Heine and K. Caparella, "Sect Kids Face Lives of Peril: Measles Isn't Only Likely Illness," *Philadelphia Daily News*, February 20, 1991.

104 **Schools cancel trips to Philadelphia:** K. Heine and K. Sheehan, "Measles Hysteria Rampant: Officials Say Fears Aren't Warranted," *Philadelphia Daily News*, February 21, 1991.

104–105 **Reverend Reinert reacts to criticism:** J. P. Blake, "'Cult' Image Disturbing: Media Seen As Fueling Public Misunderstanding," *Philadelphia Daily News*, February 22, 1991.

105 **Financial burden on Philadelphia due to measles epidemic:** R. Palley, "State Hails City's War on Measles: Will Send Extra 100G," *Philadelphia Daily News*, February 22, 1991; K. Sheehan, "Faith Tabernacle School Can Reopen, Officials Say," *Philadelphia Daily News*, February 26, 1991.

105–106 **Jacobson case:** *Jacobson v. Massachusetts*, 197 U.S. 11 (1905).

106 **Zucht case:** *Zucht v. King*, 260 U.S. 174 (1922).

106 **Parents argue religious exemption to vaccination unsuccessfully:** *Wright V. Dewitt School District*, 238 Ark. 906, 385 S.W.2d 644 (Ark. 1965); *McCartney v. Austin*, 31 A.D.2d 370, 298 N.Y.S.2d 26 (3d Dep't 1969); *Avard v. Manchester Board of School Committee et al.*, 376 F. Supp. 479 (1974).

106 **New York State bill allowing religious exemption to vaccination:** Colgrove, *State of Immunity*, 181.

107 **Polio outbreak in Christian Science school:** Centers for Disease Control and Prevention, "Follow-Up on Poliomyelitis," *Morbidity and Mortality Weekly Report* 21 (1972): 365–366; F. M. Foote, G. Kraus, M. D. Andrews, and J. C. Hart, "Polio Outbreak in a Private School," *Connecticut Medicine*, December 1973.

107 **Health official responds to polio outbreak:** S. W. Ferguson, "Mandatory Immunization," *New England Journal of Medicine* 288 (1973): 800.

107 **Philadelphia mayor Wilson Goode regarding obtaining court order requiring measles vaccinations:** H. Goldman and S. Fitzgerald, "City Will Seek Court Order for Measles Shots," *Philadelphia Inquirer*, February 28, 1991.

108 **CDC's Dr. William Atkinson regarding court order:** H. Goldman and S. Fitzgerald, "Measles Ruling Questioned: Goes Far Beyond What City Asked," *Philadelphia Inquirer*, March 6, 1991.

108 **Reverend Reinert claims persecution:** H. Goldman, "ACLU Declines to Help Parents in Measles Case," *Philadelphia Inquirer*, March 2, 1991.

109 **ACLU of Florida:** H. Daniels, "ACLU Files Suit Over 'Devil' Shirts," *The Gainesville Sun*, November 24, 2009.

109 **ACLU of Eastern Missouri:** "ACLU of Eastern Missouri Challenges Law Banning Pickets and Protests One Hour Before or After Funeral," http://www.aclu.org/freespeech/protest/26265prs20060721.html.

109 **Nazis in Skokie:** E. Grabianowski, "How the ACLU Works," http://people.howstuffworks.com/aclu3.htm/printable.

109 **ACLU satirized:** "ACLU Defends Nazi's Right to Burn Down ACLU Headquarters," *The Onion*, October 14, 2003.

109 **ACLU refuses to take parents' case:** H. Goldman, "ACLU Declines to Help Parents in Measles Case," *Philadelphia Inquirer*, March 2, 1991.

110 **Judge Edward Summers orders vaccination:** H. Goldman, "Judge Permits City to Vaccinate Objectors," *Philadelphia Inquirer*, March 5, 1991; K. Sheehan and D. L. Figueroa, "Another Child Dies of Measles," *Philadelphia Daily News*, March 8, 1991.

111 **Judge Vincent Cirillo's ruling on vaccination appeal; James Jones's death:** J. O'Dowd, "Measles Heartbreak: Stricken Baby on Life Support: Measles Fear: Tot 'Critical,'" *Philadelphia Daily News*, March 7, 1991; K. Sheehan and D. L. Figueroa, "Another Child Dies of Measles," *Philadelphia Daily News*, March 8, 1991; H. Goldman, "Church Child Dies," *Philadelphia Inquirer*, March 9, 1991; K. Sheehan, "5 Children Get Shots: Court Ordered Vaccinations," *Philadelphia Daily News*, March 9, 1991.

111 **Health Commissioner Ross vaccinates Faith Tabernacle Congregation children:** H. Goldman, "Church Child Dies," *Philadelphia Inquirer*, March 9, 1991.

111 **Second round of inoculations and lawyer James Balter's decision not to oppose them:** H. Goldman, "Inoculations Ordered in 3 More Cases," *Philadelphia Inquirer*, March 15, 1991.

111–112 **Robert Levenson, director of Philadelphia's division of disease control, regarding outbreak subsiding:** S. Fitzgerald, "Measles Epidemic Slows," *Philadelphia Inquirer*, June 7, 1991.

112 **Reverend Reinert on rewards of faith:** J. P. Blake, "'Cult' Image Disturbing: Media Seen As Fueling Public Misunderstanding," *Philadelphia Daily News*, February 22, 1991.

112 **CDC report:** D. V. Rodgers, J. S. Gindler, W. L. Atkinson, and L. E. Markowitz, "High Attack Rates and Case Fatality During a Measles Outbreak in Groups with Religious Exemption to Vaccination," *Pediatric Infectious Disease Journal* 12 (1993): 288–92.

112 **Number of children unimmunized in US for religious reasons:** Centers for Disease Control and Prevention, "Vaccination Coverage Among Children in Kindergarten—United States, 2012–2013 School Year," *Morbidity and Mortality Weekly Report* 62 (2013): 607–612.

Chapter 8: Ungodly Acts

113 **Gary and Margaret Hall:** *Hall v. State*, 493 N.E.2d 433 (Ind. 1986).

114 **Jesus's views regarding illness not those of his faith:** Kelsey, *Healing Christianity*, 52.

114 **Jesus influenced by Book of Job:** Ibid., 35.

117–118 **Dr. Jack Provonsha regarding Jesus as the Father of Modern Medicine:** Kelsey, *Healing Christianity*, 329.

118 **Jesus's acceptance of doctors:** Ibid., 78 (italics added).

118 **Morton Kelsey regarding illness as a test of faith:** Ibid., 76–77.

119 **Polycarp, Bishop of Smyrna, regarding Christian responsibility for the sick:** Porterfield, *Healing in the History of Christianity*, 5.

119 **Amanda Porterfield regarding early Christians:** Ibid., 47.

119 **Christian monasteries as forerunners of hospitals:** Crislip, *Monastery to Hospital*, 9–38.

119 **Christian hospitals in the Middle Ages:** Porterfield, *Healing in the History of Christianity*, 76.

119 **Missionary interest in modern medicine:** Ibid., 141.

119 **Work of Dr. Albert Schweitzer:** Brabazon, *Schweitzer*, 241–242, 338–339; Schweitzer, *Out of My Life and Thought*, 137.

119 **United Church Mission Hospitals:** Burrows, *Healing in the Wilderness*.

119–120   **Edward Bliss and missionaries in China:** Porterfield, *Healing in the History of Christianity*, 152–157.

120   **Religious-based health care in the United States:** "Religious Hospitals, Mergers, and Refusal Clauses," Law Students for Reproductive Justice, 2008; C. Price, "Hospitals—A Historical Perspective," *Clearly Caring Magazine*, 27 (2007).

120   **Gezer excavations:** Payne, *Child in Human Progress*, 150.

121   **Ta'Annek excavations:** Ibid., 152

121   **Jericho:** Bakan, *Slaughter*, 29.

121   **Universality of infanticide:** Payne, *Child in Human Progress*, 152.

121   **Manner in which children were killed in ancient times:** deMause, *History of Childhood*, 17, 25, 32; Breiner, *Slaughter*, 6, 16.

121   **Ancient boys used in love potions:** Breiner, *Slaughter*, 117.

121   **Ancient children beaten for nightmares:** Ibid., 115.

121   **Ancient children used for entertainment:** Ibid., 120.

121   **Ancient children sacrificed for Diocletian:** Ibid., 117–118.

121   **Infanticide as population control:** Ibid., 8.

121   **Ancient children most likely to be sacrificed:** Payne, *Child in Human Progress*, 150–151; Breiner, *Slaughter*, 7–8.

121   **Burying daughters:** Payne, *Child in Human Progress*, 171–172.

121–122   **Male predominance as a consequence of female infanticide:** deMause, *History of Childhood*, 26.

122   **Abraham saved by Gabriel:** Bakan, *Slaughter of the Innocents*, 28

122   **The valley of Hinnom turned into a garbage dump:** Ibid., 28–29.

123   **Plato and Aristotle supported killing deformed children:** Ibid., 31; deMause, *History of Childhood*, 26.

123   **Seneca regarding mutilating children:** Breiner, *Slaughter*, 111; Payne, *Child in Human Progress*, 243.

123   **William Lecky regarding infanticide in the Roman Empire:** Bakan, *Slaughter of the Innocents*, 31–32.

123   **Hippocrates and sexual abuse of children:** Helfer, *Battered Child*, 11.

124   ***London Bridge Is Falling Down:*** deMause, *History of Childhood*, 27; Bakan, *Slaughter of the Innocents*, 63–64.

124   ***Hush-a-bye Baby:*** Bakan, *Slaughter of the Innocents*, 60.

124   ***Ladybird, Ladybird, Fly Away Home:*** Ibid., 63.

124   **Punch and Judy:** Ibid., 68.

125   **Abandonment allowed ancient parents to claim they hadn't committed infanticide:** Breiner, *Slaughter*, 9.

126   **History of childhood is a nightmare:** Helfer, *Battered Child*, 6.

127   **Constantine's edict in AD 315:** Payne, *Child in Human Progress*, 264–265.

127   **Christian teachings influenced barbarian tribes:** deMause, *History of Childhood*, 90.

127   **Constantine's edict in AD 321:** Payne, *Child in Human Progress*, 265.

127   **Payne regarding early Christians and child welfare:** Ibid., 258.

Chapter 9: The Miracle Business

131   **Arpad Vass's cadaver studies:** Roach, Mary. *Stiff: The Curious Lives of Cadavers*. New York: W. W. Norton and Company, 2004, 61–84.

131–132   **Christian healing:** Porterfield, *Healing in the History of Christianity*, 50–51.

132   **Richard Sloan regarding relationship between religion and magic:** Sloan, *Blind Faith*, 21.

133   **List of saints and what they cure:** Rose, *Faith Healing*, 34.

133   **Christopher Pick regarding saints and relics:** Pick, *Miracles of the World*, 102.

133–134   **List of relics:** Randi, *Faith Healers*, 30; Nickell, *Looking for a Miracle*, 73–76; Finucane, *Miracles and Pilgrims*, 31.

134   **Vigilantius of Talouse objects to relics:** Nickell, *Looking for a Miracle*, 74.

134   **Pope Innocent III recognizes legitimacy of healing orders centered on saints and relics:** Rose, *Faith Healing*, 34.

134   **Pope Innocent III orders verification of relics:** Finucane, *Miracles and Pilgrims*, 31.

134–135   **The royal touch:** Randi, *Faith Healers*, 31; Rose, *Faith Healing*, 35–38.

135   **Martin Luther regarding miracles:** Porterfield, *Healing in the History of Christianity*, 23–25.

135   **Luther regarding miracles:** Kelsey, *Healing Christianity*, 173–174.

135–136   **The story of Bernadette Soubirous:** Cranston, *Lourdes*, 8–11; Randi, *Faith Healers*, 36–40; Nickell, *Looking for a Miracle*, 145–153; Rose, *Faith Healing*, 93.

136   **The Shrine at Lourdes:** Randi, *Faith Healers*, 37; Nickell, *Looking for a Miracle*, 152.

137   **A day at Lourdes:** Frank, *Persuasion and Healing*, 55–56.

137   **Pilgrim regarding visit to Lourdes:** Ibid., 56.

137   **Archbishop of Canterbury regarding faith healing:** Rose, *Faith Healing*, 176.

137   **Lutheran Church regarding faith healing:** Randi, *Faith Healers*, 85.

137–138   **Church of Canada regarding faith healing:** Ibid., 72–73.

138   **Prospero Lambertini and the Roman Catholic Church regarding faith healing:** Nickell, *Looking for a Miracle*, 10–11.

138   **Reverend George Johnstone Jeffrey regarding faith healing:** Rose, *Faith Healing*, 177.

138   **Oral Roberts:** Randi, *Faith Healers*, 241–258, 370–371.

139   **Peter Popoff:** Ibid., 187–239; Nickell, *Looking for a Miracle*, 137–139.

139–140   **Pat Robertson:** Randi, *Faith Healers*, 257–267.

140–141   **Jim Bakker:** http://en.wikipedia.org/wiki/Jim_Bakker; Nickell, *Looking for a Miracle*, 102.

141   **Jimmy Swaggart:** http://en.wikipedia.org/wiki/Jimmy_Swaggart.

141–142   **Tony Campolo regarding Pentecostalism:** Campolo, *How to Be a Pentecostal without Speaking in Tongues*, 23.

142–143   **Fabrizio Benedetti pain experiment:** M. Amanzio, A. Pollo, G. Maggi, and F. Benedetti, "Response Variability to Analgesics: A Role for Non-Specific Activation of Endogenous Opioids," *Pain* 90 (2001): 205–215.

143   **Parkinson's disease study:** R. Fuente-Fernández, T. J. Ruth, V. Sossi, et al., "Expectation and Dopamine Release: Mechanism of the Placebo Effect in Parkinson's Disease," *Science* 293 (2001): 1164–1166.

143   **Learning to enhance or suppress the immune system:** M. E. E. Sabbioni, D. H. Bovbjerg, S. Mathew, et al., "Classically Conditioned Changes in Plasma Cortisol Levels Induced by Dexamethasone in Healthy Men," *FASEB Journal* 11 (1997): 1291–1296; D. L. Longo, P. L. Duffy, W. C. Koop, et al., "Conditioned Immune Response to Interferon-Gamma in Humans," *Clinical Immunology* 90 (1999): 173–181.

143   **Asthma study:** M. E. Wechsler, J. M. Kelley, I. O. E. Boyd, et al., "Active Albuterol or Placebo, Sham Acupuncture, or No Intervention in Asthma," *New England Journal of Medicine* 365 (2011): 119–126.

143   **Knee surgery study:** J. B. Moseley, K. O'Malley, N. J. Petersen, et al., "A Controlled Trial of Arthroscopic Surgery for Osteoarthritis of the Knee," *New England Journal of Medicine* 347 (2002): 81–88.

Chapter 10: The Peculiar People

146–147   **Trials of the Peculiar People:** Peters, *When Prayer Fails*, 49–66.

148   **Emma Judd case:** Ibid., 76–77.

148–149   **Luther Pierson case:** Ibid., 78–81.

149–150   **Adell Sherbert case:** *Sherbert v. Verner*, 374 U.S. 398 (1963).

150   **Amish parents case:** *Wisconsin v. Yoder*, 406 U.S. 205, 215 (1972).

150–151   **Ohio prisoners case:** *Cutter v. Wilkinson*, 544 U.S. 709, 718–719 (2005); A. Johnson, "Court Upholds Religious Prisoners' Rights," www.msnbc.msn.com/id/8047388/#.UIOSdrT9Llo.

151–154   **Santeria case:** D. O'Brien, *Animal Sacrifice and Religious Freedom*; Church of the Lukumi Babalu Aye, Inc. v. City of Hialeah, 508 U.S. 520 (1993).

154–155   **Sarah Prince case:** *Prince v. Commonwealth of Massachusetts*, 321 U.S. 158.

155–156   **George Reynolds case:** *Reynolds v. United States*, 98 U.S. 145.

156   **George Cannon regarding the George Reynolds case:** G. O. Larson, "Federal Government Efforts to 'Americanize' Utah Before Admission to Statehood," J. Willard Marriott Library, University of Utah.

156–157   **Alfred Smith and Galen Black case regarding Native Americans and peyote:** Long, *Religious Freedom and Indian Rights*.

158   **Jehovah's Witnesses' beliefs:** Peters, *When Prayer Fails*, 167.

158   **Cheryl Linn Labrenz case:** *People ex rel. Wallace v. Labrenz*, 104 N.E. 2d 769 (Ill. 1952).

158   **Joseph Perricone case:** *State v. Perricone*, 181 A.2d 751 (N.J. 1962).

158   **Soto twins case:** *In the matter of the Guardianship of L. S. and H. S.*, 87 P.3d 521 (Nev. 2004).

158–159   **Willimina Anderson case:** *Raleigh Fitkin-Paul Morgan Memorial Hospital v. Anderson*, 201 A.2d 537 (N.J. 1964); M. Illson, "Pregnant Woman May Not Need Transfusion Ordered by Court," *New York Times*, June 21, 1964.

159   **Jesse Jones case:** *Application of the Presidents and Directors of Georgetown College*, 331 F.2d 1000 (D.C. Cir. 1964).

159   **United States Supreme Court hears Jehovah's Witnesses case:** *Jehovah's Witnesses v. King County Hospital*, 390 U.S. 598 (1968).

160–161   **The Hobby Lobby decision:** *Hobby Lobby v. Sebelius*, 568 U.S., 2012; A. Liptak, "Supreme Court Rejects Contraceptives Mandate for Some Corporations," *New York Times*, June 30, 2014; J. Levs, "What the Supreme Court's Hobby Lobby Decision Means," *CNN*, June 30, 2014; I. Carmon, "The Hobby Lobby Decision Isn't Narrow," *MSNBC*, June 30, 2014; J. Gerstein and D. Nather, "Hobby Lobby Decision: 5 Takeaways,"

Politico, June 30, 2014; D. Marbury, "Will the Hobby Lobby Decision Allow Employers to Ignore Medical Evidence?" *Medical Economics*, July 1, 2014; D. Reiss, "Hobby Lobby and Religious Exemptions: The Good, the Bad, and the Ugly," *Skeptical Raptor*, July 1, 2014, www.skepticalraptor.com/skepticalraptorblog.php/hobby-lobby-religious-exemptions-good-bad-ugly.

Chapter 11: The Divine Whisper

163–165   **Mary Ellen:** Riis, *Children of the Poor*, 91–96; Nelson, *Making an Issue of Child Abuse*, 7–9; Helfer, *Battered Child*, 17; Heimlich, *Breaking Their Will*, 40; Payne, *Child in Human Progress*, 335–336; Coleman, *Human Society Leaders in America*, 38–76.

165   **Forms of child abuse:** C. Flato, "Parents Who Beat Children," *Saturday Evening Post*, October 6, 1962.

165   **The Society for the Prevention of Cruelty to Children:** Payne, *Child in Human Progress*, 335–336; Coleman, *Human Society Leaders in America*, 38–76.

166   **John Caffey's first paper:** J. Caffey and W. A. Silverman, "Infantile Cortical Hyperostosis: Preliminary Report of a New Syndrome," *American Journal of Roentgenology*, 54 (1945): 1.

166   **Caffey's second paper:** J. Caffey, "Multiple Fractures in the Long Bones of Infants Suffering from Chronic Subdural Hematoma," *American Journal of Roentgenology*, 56 (1946): 163–173.

166–167   **Fred Silverman's paper:** F. N. Silverman, "The Roentgen Manifestations of Unrecognized Skeletal Trauma in Infants," *American Journal of Roentgenology*, 69 (1953): 413–427 (italics added).

167   **Henry Kempe's paper:** C. H. Kempe, F. N. Silverman, B. F. Steele, et al., "The Battered Child Syndrome," *Journal of the American Medical Association*, 181 (1962): 17–24.

167   **"Parents Who Beat Children":** C. Flato, "Parents Who Beat Children," *Saturday Evening Post*, October 6, 1962.

167–168   **Response to Kempe's paper:** Nelson, *Making an Issue of Child Abuse*, 61–63.

168   **Jolly K's testimony at Mondale hearings:** Child Abuse Prevention and Treatment Act, 1973. Hearings Before the Subcommittee on Children and Youth of the Committee on Labor and Public Welfare, United States Senate,

Ninety-Third Congress, First Session on S.1191, 49–59; Nelson, *Making an Issue of Child Abuse*, 105.

168–169 **Child Abuse Prevention and Treatment Act, creation and impact:** Nelson, *Making an Issue of Child Abuse*, 1–2, 100–117; Mason, *Father's Property to Children's Rights*, 150.

169–170 **Lisa Sheridan case:** Fraser, *God's Perfect Child*, 279–284; Peters, *When Prayer Fails*, 113–115; Schoepflin, *Christian Science on Trial*, 202–203.

171 **Influence of Christian Scientists on CAPTA:** Rita Swan, personal communication, January 29, 2014.

171 **States add religious exemptions to CAPTA:** Fraser, *God's Perfect Child*, 284–285; Peters, *When Prayer Fails*, 116.

171–172 **Amy Hermanson case:** J. C. Merrick, "Spiritual Healing, Sick Kids and the Law: Inequities in the American Healthcare System," 29 Am. J. L. & Med. 269: 18–19.

172 **2013 religious exemptions from child abuse and neglect laws:** *Children's Healthcare Is a Legal Duty*, www.childrenshealthcare.org.

172 **Religious exemptions from child abuse and neglect laws of no benefit:** J. C. Merrick, "Spiritual Healing, Sick Kids and the Law: Inequities in the American Healthcare System," 29 Am. J. L. & Med. 269: 14.

173–176 **Sarah Hershberger case:** A. Kumar, "Ohio Hospital Fights Amish Girl's Refusal to Continue Chemotherapy," *Christian Post*, August 26, 2013; J. Seewer, "Ohio Hospital: Force Amish Girl to Have Chemo," *Associated Press*, August 23, 2013; J. Seewer, "Court Sides with Ohio Hospital on Amish Care," *Associated Press*, August 28, 2013; J. Seewer, "Judge Again Blocks Ohio Hospital's Attempt to Force Amish Girl to Resume Cancer Treatments," *Associated Press*, September 4, 2013; J. Seewer, "Judge Blocks Bid to Force Amish Girl to Have Chemo," *Associated Press*, September 5, 2013; J. Seewer, "Amish Family Flees to Avoid Chemotherapy," *Associated Press*, November 28, 2013; S. Goldstein, "Amish Girl in Hiding to Avoid Ohio Court's Ruling on Her Cancer Treatment Options," *New York Daily News*, November 29, 2013; L. Tillson, "Amish Girl with Cancer Forced to Go into Hiding to Avoid Chemotherapy Treatments," *National Monitor*, November 30, 2013; S. Goldstein, "Amish Girl in Hiding to Avoid Ohio Court's Ruling on Her Cancer Treatment Options," *New York Daily News*, November 29, 2013; "Guardian Ends Bid to Force Amish Girl Into Chemo," *Associated Press*, February 14, 2014; C. Moraff, "In the Death of a Child, the Interests of the State Eclipse Parental Rights," http://blog.pennlive.com/opinion/print

.html?entry=/2014/02/in_the_death_of_a_child_the_in.html., February 23, 2014.

174–175 **Fourteenth Amendment and school integration:** G. Engle, "Towards a New Lens of Analysis: The History and Future of Religious Exemptions to Child Neglect Statutes," 14 Rich. J. L. & Pub. Int. 375: 5.

175 **Fourteenth Amendment and children's rights:** R. Swan, "On Statutes Depriving a Class of Children of Rights to Medical Care: Can this Discrimination Be Litigated?" 2 Quinnipiac Health L. J. 73 1998–1999: 94.

175 **Seth Miskimens case:** *Ohio v. Miskimens*, 490 N.E.2d 931, 935–936 (Ohio Ct. Com. Pl. 1984).

Chapter 12: Standing Up

177–178 **Rita Swan visits Wayne State University Medical Library:** Interview with Rita Swan, June 17, 2013.

178–180 **Rita and Doug Swan on Donohue:** *The Phil Donohue Show*, November 1979.

179 **Rita Swan regarding letters:** *Kelly and Company, WXYZ*, Detroit, May 1982, *ABC TV*.

180 **Rita Swan regarding friends:** Interview with Rita Swan, June 17, 2013.

180 **Rita Swan regarding societal responsibility:** *Crossroads* with Charles Kurault and Bill Moyers, CBS Network, June 27, 1984; *Nightline* with Ted Koppel, *ABC TV*, June 17, 1988.

180 **Asser/Swan study:** S. M. Asser and R. Swan, "Child Fatalities from Religion-Motivated Medical Neglect," *Pediatrics* 101 (1998): 625–629.

180–181 **Medical examiner regarding puerperal sepsis:** R. Swan, "Yet Another Follower's Child Harmed by Medical Neglect," *Children's Healthcare Is a Legal Duty* newsletter, Number 2, 2010.

181 **Deaths from bloodstream infections, pneumonia, and meningitis:** Peters, *When Prayer Fails*, 16.

181 **Seth Asser regarding unreported and misreported faith healing deaths:** Peters, *When Prayer Fails*, 14.

183 **Other groups supporting removal of religious exemptions from child abuse and neglect laws:** Peters, *When Prayer Fails*, 15; J. C. Merrick, "Spiritual Healing, Sick Kids and the Law: Inequities in the American Healthcare System," 29 Am. J. L. & Med. 269: 8.

183   **Five states eliminate religious exemptions from child abuse laws:** *Children's Healthcare Is a Legal Duty*, www.childrenshealthcare.org.

183   **Prosecutor on futility of prosecuting religious exemption cases:** Peters, *When Prayer Fails*, 14.

183   **Freud and religious zealotry:** D. Williams, "Punishing the Faithful: Freud, Religion, and the Law," 24 Cardozo L. Rev. 2181: 2.

184   **Christian Scientists believe legislators support faith healing:** A. Dose, "Government Endorsement of Living on a Prayer," 30 J. Legal Med. 515: 2.

184   **Rita Swan and David Twitchell regarding respect for the law:** Interview with Rita Swan, June 17, 2013.

184   **Twitchell regarding doing things differently:** *NBC Channel 30*, Hartford, Connecticut, "To Die for the Faith," April 1999.

184   **Absence of religious exemptions to child abuse and neglect laws in Canada and Great Britain:** J. C. Merrick, "Spiritual Healing, Sick Kids and the Law: Inequities in the American Healthcare System," 29 Am. J. L. & Med. 269: 2.

185   **Lack of concern regarding child deaths in Oregon:** Interview with Rita Swan, June 17, 2013.

185   **Terry Gustafson regarding problems with the law and child deaths in Oregon:** *ABC News 20/20*, May 6, 1988.

185   **Followers of Christ Church's child deaths:** *Channel 2*, Oregon, "Too Much Religious Freedom," April 1998, *ABC TV*.

185   **Response among members of the Followers of Christ Church to the Starr bill:** Peters, *When Prayer Fails*, 199; R. Swan, "Followers Sentenced to Long Prison Term in Baby's Death," *Children's Healthcare Is a Legal Duty* newsletter, Number 4, 2011; "Rita's AAP Acceptance Speech," http://childrenshealthcare .org/?page_id=1037.

187   **Followers of Christ Church members in Oregon move to Idaho, where death rates among children are high:** Rita Swan, personal communications, November 10, 2013 and January 31, 2014.

187–188   **Jerry Sandusky case:** "Summary of the Investigation and the Charges Against the Former Penn State University Defensive Coordinator," *York Daily Record*, July 8, 2012; Freeh, Sporkin & Sullivan, LLP, "Report of the Special Investigative Counsel of The Penn State University Related to Child Sexual Abuse Committed by Gerald A. Sandusky," July 12, 2012.

189   **Pennsylvania considers tightening child abuse laws:** The General Assembly of Pennsylvania, Senate Bills No. 20 and 28, introduced March 15, 2013.

189   **The Schaible case:** M. Newall, "Couple Probed in Death of 2d Child," *Philadelphia Inquirer*, April 20, 2013; M. Newall, "Second Ill Child of Devout Parents Dies," *Philadelphia Inquirer*, April 23, 2013; M. Newall, "Schaibles' Oversight Was Issue in 2011," *Philadelphia Inquirer*, April 24, 2013; M. Newall, "Pastor: 'Spiritual Lack' Killed Two Boys, *Philadelphia Inquirer*, April 28, 2013; M. Newall, "Death of Faith-Healing Couple's Baby Is Ruled Homicide," *Philadelphia Inquirer*, May 22, 2013; S. Leach, "M. E.: Death of Faith-Healing Couple's Baby Is Murder," *Philadelphia Daily News*, May 22, 2013; M. Dribben, "Schaible Couple Denied Release," *Philadelphia Inquirer*, May 25, 2013; "Pennsylvania Religious Objectors Lose a Second Baby," *Children's Healthcare Is a Legal Duty* newsletter, Number 1, 2013.

189–191   **The Schaibles are convicted and sentenced:** J. A. Slobodzian, "No-Contest Plea by Parents in Faith-Healing Death of 2d Child," *Philadelphia Inquirer*, November 16, 2013; J. A. Slobodzian, "Judge Sends Schaibles to Prison," *Philadelphia Inquirer*, February 20, 2014.

191   **Rita Swan fights Pennsylvania's religious exemptions to medical neglect laws:** R. Swan, personal communication, June 14, 2013.

193   **Why Americans haven't opposed religious exemptions to medical care:** S. St. Amand, "Protecting Neglect: The Constitutionality of Spiritual Healing Exemptions to Child Protection Statutes," 12 Rich. J. L. & Pub. Int. 139:5.

Epilogue: "The Frail Web of Understanding"

195   **Rita Swan's acceptance speech:** "AAP President Recognizes Dr. Swan for Work on Children's Equal Rights to Health Care," *AAP News*, volume 33, May 2012; "Rita's AAP Acceptance Speech," http://childrenshealth care.org/?page_id=1037.

196   **Getting past the guilt:** *Crossroads* with Charles Kurault and Bill Moyers, June 27, 1984, *CBS Network*.

197   **Rita Swan regarding humanity:** Interview with author, May 22, 2013.

197   **Erich Fromm regarding man's relationship to God:** Fromm, *Escape From Freedom*, 139–140.

SELECTED BIBLIOGRAPHY

Alarcón, Renato D. and Frank, Julia B. *The Psychotherapy of Hope: The Legacy of Persuasion and Healing*. Baltimore: Johns Hopkins University Press, 2012.

American Psychiatric Association. *Diagnostic and Statistical Manual of Mental Disorders: Fifth Edition, DSM-5*. Washington, D.C.: American Psychiatric Publishing, 2013.

Arendt, Hannah. *Eichmann in Jerusalem: A Report on the Banality of Evil*. New York: Viking Press, 1963.

Aslan, Reza. *Zealot: The Life and Times of Jesus of Nazareth*. New York: Random House, 2013.

Bakan, David. *Slaughter of the Innocents: A Study of the Battered Child Phenomenon*. San Francisco: Jossey-Bass Publishers, 1979.

Blass, Thomas. *The Man Who Shocked the World: The Life and Legacy of Stanley Milgram*. New York: Basic Books, 2004.

Boonin, David. *A Defense of Abortion*. Cambridge: Cambridge University Press, 2003.

Brabazon, James. *Albert Schweitzer*. Syracuse: Syracuse University Press, 2000.

Breiner, Sander J. *Slaughter of the Innocents: Child Abuse Through the Ages and Today*. New York: Plenum Press, 1990.

Burrows, Bob. *Healing in the Wilderness: A History of the United Church Mission Hospitals*. Madeira Park, British Columbia: Harbour Publishing Co., 2004.

Cather, W., Milmine, G., Stouck, D. *Mary Baker G. Eddy & the History of Christian Science*. New York: Doubleday, Page & Co., 1909.

Cavender, Anthony. *Folk Medicine in Southern Appalachia*. Chapel Hill: The University of North Carolina Press, 2003.

Coleman, Sydney H. *Human Society Leaders in America*. Albany: The American Humane Association, 1924.

Colgrove, James. *State of Immunity: The Politics of Vaccination in Twentieth-Century America*. Berkeley: University of California Press, 2006.

Compolo, Tony. *How to Be a Pentecostal Without Speaking in Tongues*. Dallas, Texas: Word Publishing, 1991.

Cranston, Ruth. *The Miracle of Lourdes*. New York: McGraw-Hill Book Company, Inc., 1955.

Crislip, Andrew T. *From Monastery to Hospital: Christian Monasticism & the Transformation of Health Care in Late Antiquity*. Ann Arbor: The University of Michigan Press, 2005.

deMause, Lloyd. *The History of Childhood*. Northvale, New Jersey: Jason Aronson, Inc., 1974.

Dobbert, Duane L. *Understanding Personality Disorders*. Lanham, Maryland: Rowman & Littlefield, 2007.

Dombrowski, Daniel A., Deltete, R. J. *A Brief, Liberal, Catholic Defense of Abortion*. Urbana, Illinois: University of Illinois Press, 2000.

Eddy, Mary Baker. *Science and Health with Key to the Scriptures*. Boston: The Christian Science Board of Directors, 2000.

Finucane, Ronald C. *Miracles and Pilgrims: Popular Beliefs in Medieval England*. New York: St. Martin's Press, 1977.

Frank, Jerome D. *Persuasion and Healing*. New York: Schocken Books, 1961.

Fraser, Carolyn. *God's Perfect Child: Living and Dying in the Christian Science Church*. New York: Henry Holt and Company, 1999.

Fromm, Erich. *Escape from Freedom*. New York: Henry Holt and Company, 1941.

———. *The Sane Society*. New York: Fawcett World Library, 1955.

———. *The Anatomy of Human Destructiveness*. New York: Henry Holt and Company, 1973.

Groopman, Jerome. *The Anatomy of Hope: How People Prevail in the Face of Illness*. New York: Random House, 2004.

Hamilton, Marci A. *God vs. the Gavel: Religion and the Rule of Law*. Cambridge: Cambridge University Press, 2005.

———. *Justice Denied: What America Must Do to Protect Its Children*. Cambridge: Cambridge University Press, 2008.

Heimlich, Janet. *Breaking Their Will: Shedding Light on Religious Child Maltreatment*. Amherst, New York: Prometheus Books, 2011.

Helfer, Mary Edna, Kempe, Ruth S., Krugman, Richard D. (eds.). *The Battered Child*. Fifth Edition. Chicago: The University of Chicago Press, 1997.

Hoffer, Eric. *The True Believer: Thoughts on the Nature of Mass Movements*. New York: HarperPerennial, 1951.

Hood, Fred J. *The Religious Right vs. Right Religion: A Biblical Critique of Conservative Religious Imperialism*. Wyoming, Michigan: Principia Media, 2012.

Jenny, Carole. *Child Abuse and Neglect: Diagnosis, Treatment, and Evidence*. St. Louis: Elsevier Saunders, 2011.

Jensen, David H. *Graced Vulnerability: A Theology of Childhood*. Cleveland: The Pilgrim Press, 2005.

Kelsey, Morton. *Healing and Christianity*. Minneapolis: Augsburg Fortress, 1995.

Klusendorf, Scott. *The Case for Life: Equipping Christians to Engage the Culture*. Wheaton, Illinois: Crossway, 2009.

Koenig, Harold G., McConnell, Malcolm. *The Healing Power of Faith: How Belief and Prayer Can Help You Triumph Over Disease*. New York: Touchstone, 1999.

———. *Spirituality in Patient Care: Why, How, When, and What*. West Conshohocken, Pennsylvania: Templeton Press, 2007.

———. *Medicine, Religion, and Health: Where Science and Spirituality Meet*. West Conshohocken, Pennsylvania: Templeton Foundation Press, 2008.

———. *Spirituality & Health Research: Methods, Measurement, Statistics, and Resources*. West Conshohocken, Pennsylvania: Templeton Foundation Press, 2011.

Kramer, Linda S. *The Religion that Kills: Christian Science: Abuse, Neglect, and Mind Control*. Lafayette, Louisiana: Huntington House Press, 2000.

Levin, Jeff. *God, Faith, and Health: Exploring the Spirituality-Healing Connection*. New York: John Wiley & Sons, Inc., 2001.

Lifton, Robert J. *Thought Reform and the Psychology of Totalism: A Study of 'Brainwashing' in China*. Chapel Hill: The University of North Carolina Press, 1989.

———. *Witness to an Extreme Century: A Memoir*. New York: Free Press, 2011.

Linedecker, Clifford L. *Massacre at Waco: The Shocking True Story of Cult Leader David Koresh and the Branch Davidians*. London: True Crime, 1993.

Long, Carolyn N. *Religious Freedom and Indian Rights: The Case of Oregon v. Smith*. Lawrence: University Press of Kansas, 2000.

Lunt, Peter. *Stanley Milgram: Understanding Obedience and Its Implications*. New York: Palgrave Macmillan, 2009.

Mason, Mary Ann. *From Father's Property to Children's Rights: The History of Child Custody in the United States*. New York: Columbia University Press, 1994.

Matthews, Dale A., Clark, Connie. *The Faith Factor: Proof of the Healing Power of Prayer*. New York: Penguin, 1998.

Milgram, Stanley. *Obedience to Authority*. New York: Harper & Row Publishers, 1974.

Nelson, Barbara J. *Making an Issue of Child Abuse: Political Agenda Setting for Social Problems*. Chicago: The University of Chicago Press, 1984.

Nickell, Joe. *Looking for a Miracle: Weeping Icons, Relics, Stigmata, Visions & Healing Cures*. Amherst, New York: Prometheus Books, 1998.

Nolen, William A. *Healing: A Doctor in Search of a Miracle*. New York: Random House, 1974.

O'Brien, David M. *Animal Sacrifice and Religious Freedom: Church of the Lukumi Babalu Aye v. City of Hialeah*. Lawrence: University Press of Kansas, 2004.

O'Brien, George Dennis. *The Church and Abortion: A Catholic Dissent*. Lanham, Maryland: The Rowman & Littlefield Publishing Group, 2010.

Parker, Larry. *We Let Our Son Die: A Parents' Search for Truth*. Irvine, California: Harvest House Publishers, 1980.

———. *No Spin Faith: Rejecting Religious Spin Doctors*. Mustang, Oklahoma: Tate Publishing, 2007.

Payne, George Henry. *The Child in Human Progress*. New York: G. P. Putnam's Sons, 1912.

Perkins, Rodney, Jackson, Forrest. *Cosmic Suicide: The Tragedy and Transcendence of Heaven's Gate*. Dallas: The Pentaradial Press, 1997.

Peters, Shawn Francis. *When Prayer Fails: Faith Healing, Children, and the Law*. New York: Oxford University Press, 2008.

Pick, Christopher. *Miracles of the World*. Secaucus, New Jersey: Chartwell Books, 1929.

Pilch, John J. *Healing in the New Testament: Insights from Medical and Mediterranean Anthropology*. Minneapolis: Fortress Press, 2000.

Porterfield, Amanda. *Healing in the History of Christianity*. Oxford: Oxford University Press, 2005.

Randi, James. *The Faith Healers*. Amherst, New York: Prometheus Books, 1989.

Reitman, Janet. *Inside Scientology: The Story of America's Most Secretive Religion*. New York: Houghton Mifflin Harcourt, 2011.

Riis, Jacob. *The Children of the Poor*. New York: Charles Scribner's Sons, 1892.

Rose, Louis, Morgan, Bryan. *Faith Healing*. Harmondsworth, Middlesex, England: Penguin Books, 1968.

Scarnecchia, D. Brian. *Bioethics, Law, and Human Life Issues: A Catholic Perspective on Marriage, Family, Contraception, Abortion, Reproductive Technology, and Death and Dying*. Lanham, Maryland: The Scarecrow Press, 2010.

Scheeres, Julia. *A Thousand Lives: The Untold Story of Jonestown*. New York: Free Press, 2011.

Schoefplin, Rennie B. *Christian Science on Trial: Religious Healing in America*. Baltimore: The Johns Hopkins University Press, 2003.

Schweitzer, Albert. *Out of My Life and Thought: An Autobiography.* Baltimore: Johns Hopkins University Press, 1933.

Singer, Peter. *Rethinking Life and Death: The Collapse of Our Traditional Ethics.* New York: St. Martin's Press, 1994.

Sloan, Richard P. *Blind Faith: The Unholy Alliance of Religion and Medicine.* New York: St. Martin's Griffin, 2006.

Swan, Rita. *The Last Strawberry.* Dublin: Hag's Head Press, 1979.

Tabor, James D., Gallagher, Eugene V. *Why Waco? Cults and the Battle for Religious Freedom in America.* Berkeley: University of California Press, 1995.

Triglio, John, Brighenti, Kenneth. *Catholicism for Dummies.* Hoboken, New Jersey: John Wiley & Sons, 2012.

Wright, Lawrence. *Going Clear: Scientology, Hollywood & the Prison of Belief.* New York: Alfred A. Knopf, 2013.

Zimbardo, Philip. *The Lucifer Effect: Understanding How Good People Turn Evil.* New York: Random House, 2007.

ACKNOWLEDGMENTS

I would like to thank T. J. Kelleher for his skillful editorial hand and Gail Ross for her advocacy.

I would also like to thank Dorit Reiss, Cindy Christian, and Deborah Goodman Naisch for their help with the law; Rabbi Steve Schwartz for advice about Jewish customs and practices; Jeffrey Bergelson, Brian Fisher, Jeffrey Gerber, Janet Heimlich, Lori Kestenbaum, Jason Kim, Lois Macht, Adam Mohr, Charlotte Moser, Bonnie Offit, Carl Offit, Shirley Offit, Laura Palmer, Jason Schwartz, Alison Singer, Jake Stein, Salwa Sulieman, Kirsten Thistle, Alison Tribble, Philip Tribble, Trine Tsouderos, and Theo Zaoutis for their careful reading of the manuscript.

Most importantly, I want to acknowledge Rita Swan for being a beacon of light in a sometimes all-too-dark world.

INDEX